DR. GABE MIRKIN'S FITNESS CLINIC

DR. GABE MIRKIN'S FITNESS CLINIC

GABE MIRKIN, M.D.

CONTEMPORARY
BOOKS, INC.
CHICAGO • NEW YORK

Library of Congress Cataloging-in-Publication Data

Mirkin, Gabe.
   Dr. Gabe Mirkin's fitness clinic.

   1. Physical fitness—Miscellanea.   I. Title.
II. Title: Doctor Gabe Mirkin's fitness clinic.
[DNLM: 1. Physical Fitness—popular works. QT M675f]
GV481.M58   1986   613.7   86-6377
ISBN 0-8092-5077-2

Published by Contemporary Books, Inc.
180 North Michigan Avenue, Chicago, Illinois 60601
Manufactured in the United States of America
Library of Congress Catalog Card Number: 86-6377
International Standard Book Number: 0-8092-5077-2

Published simultaneously in Canada by Beaverbooks, Ltd.
195 Allstate Parkway, Valleywood Business Park
Markham, Ontario L3R 4T8 Canada

This book is dedicated to my wonderful children,
Gene, Jan, Jill, Geoff, and Kenneth.
They have taught me more than
I have ever learned from books.

CONTENTS

INTRODUCTION

Over the past 10 years, I have received an overwhelming number of letters from readers of my newspaper and magazine columns. An equally impressive number of questions has been collected from the audiences present at my lectures and radio call-in shows during the same time.

This book is a collection of the questions asked most frequently by athletes and aspiring athletes. It is intended to answer many of your questions, rather than to provide a comprehensive encyclopedia about sportsmedicine.

More thorough coverage of all the topics included in this book can be found in the following: *The Sportsmedicine Book* (published by Little, Brown), *Getting Thin* (published by Little, Brown), and *The Complete Sports Medicine Book for Women* (published by Simon & Schuster).

I hope that these questions and answers can save you from many of the injuries experienced by others and can help you to return to exercise as soon as possible after any injury that does occur. If you have raised some of these questions yourself, you may find it reassuring to learn that you are not alone.

If you have never exercised before, you will probably enjoy reading this book to learn what you have been missing. Hopefully, it will not be long before your own fitness program is well under way.

I hope, above all, that this book will lead you to greater enjoyment of exercise, both those activities you have practiced before and those you have not yet attempted. Perhaps your questions can inspire future generations to exercise and enjoy it.

Gabe Mirkin, M.D.

DR. GABE MIRKIN'S FITNESS CLINIC

PART I

1
WHY EXERCISE?

I am often asked why I exercise. My standard reply is that, if I saw the bus that I wanted to take pulling away, I would chase it and catch it. Exercise allows me to do things that out-of-shape people wouldn't even think of doing. I can open stuck doors and jars easily. I often run to places that I want to go and I can play basketball with the young children in the neighborhood. I would exercise even if it didn't make me more healthy. It improves the quality of my life.

Bill Emmerton, an ultramarathon runner who has twice run through Death Valley in temperatures as high as 110°F, feels the same way I do. Once he was asked what he would do if he learned that running would kill him. He replied, "I would go out and run 10 miles."

That's the way many people who regularly exercise feel about their fitness programs. But being fit does more than prepare you for physical feats. It makes you feel good and it *does* help to make you more healthy.

Read on. If you are a regular exerciser, the following pages will confirm what you know already. If you do not exercise, you will find out what you are missing.

IT MAKES YOU FEEL GOOD

Some exercises can elevate a person's mood for hours after they are performed. The more vigorous and prolonged the workout, the more likely it is that the exerciser's mood will rise.

Studies conducted at the University of Virginia by Dr. Robert S. Brown showed that intensely vigorous sports such as running and wrestling are more likely to improve a person's mood than are less demanding sports such as softball and walking.

Although this phenomenon is generally accepted by scientists and physicians, it is unclear why only certain exercises cause mood elevations. It does appear, however, that a certain minimum intensity and duration of exercise is needed. Two theories prevail: one is based on *norepinephrine*, the natural stimulant produced by the body, and the other on *endorphins*, the morphinelike chemicals the body manufactures.

It is known that depressed people have very low blood levels of norepinephrine. When these people are emotionally up, they usually have much higher levels of this chemical. It also has been shown that the norepinephrine level in a person's bloodstream rises after exercise. However, it is not known whether norepinephrine causes or just accompanies the mood elevation.

Giving endorphins to a person will improve his or her mood. But we don't know whether exercise raises the endorphin level in the brain. The only way to find this out is to take out a piece of the brain or spinal fluid during exericse. Needless to say, this has not been done.

IT HELPS YOU SLEEP AT NIGHT

Twenty-five million Americans spend more than $200 million a year on sleeping pills that don't really do them much good.

For many of these people, vigorous exercise would work much better.

In 1966 Dr. Frederick Baekland of the Downstate Medical Center in New York first demonstrated scientifically that vigorous physical exercise encourages sound, deep sleep. In more recent independent research, Dr. Colin Shapiro of Johannesburg, South Africa, and Dr. R. B. Zloty of the University of Manitoba in Canada found that the more you exercise, the more deeply you sleep.

Actively using your mind will not, in itself, encourage you to sleep. So, while studying hard for an exam or preparing a detailed report for work may make you feel tired, neither will help you to fall asleep any easier. Vigorous exercise will. Scientists are still unable to explain why.

You can, however, use exercise specifically to help you fall asleep. This is done by coordinating the times of your exercise sessions with the time you go to bed.

The most important factor in determining whether or not you will sleep is if your body temperature is dropping at that time. If you go to bed when your body temperature is rising or level, you are not likely to fall asleep.

Vigorous exercise raises your body temperature. After you finish such exercise your body temperature will remain elevated for four to six hours. If you exercise four to six hours before you go to bed, your body temperature will be dropping at bedtime.

IT HELPS KEEP YOUR BOWELS OPEN

Constipation, one of the most common complaints of young and old alike, is easily avoided by regular exercise, drinking plenty of fluids, and eating more fiber and fewer simple starches.

Infrequent bowel movements are not necessarily a sign of constipation; discomfort is. If you have infrequent bowel movements but are not uncomfortable as a result, don't worry. Although people once believed that toxic wastes build up in the colon if you don't have daily bowel movements, there is no medical evidence of this.

If you suffer from constipation, first check with your physician to make sure you are otherwise healthy. In some people, constipation may be a symptom of an obstruction of the intestines or a mineral deficiency.

Once you've found out that you're healthy, follow these tips to lessen your discomfort:

First, exercise regularly. Have you ever heard of a constipated marathon runner? There aren't any. Regular exercise increases the muscular contractions of your intestines so that food is more easily pushed along your intestinal tract.

Second, drink lots of fluids. When a stool reaches your *colon* (the lower part of your intestinal tract), water from the stool is reabsorbed into your bloodstream, hardening the stool. Drinking extra fluids will slow this process.

You should also increase your fiber intake and decrease your intake of starchy foods. Much of the refined sugar and starch that you eat is absorbed into the bloodstream, leaving very small particles that stick together in your intestines. This makes the particles difficult to pass through your intestines. However, fibrous food such as fruit, vegetables, and whole grains leaves large particles that cannot stick together in your intestines. Therefore, fiber forms bulkier, softer stools that pass easily through your intestines.

IT CLEANS YOUR BLOOD

Your bloodstream contains two chemically different types of cholesterol that perform opposite functions: a high-density one, known as *HDL*, is beneficial; a low-density one, called *LDL*, can be harmful. Exercise promotes the healthful cholesterol and cuts down on the other.

Cholesterol is not soluble, so it needs help to circulate through your bloodstream, which is comprised mainly of water. To do this your body produces a protein capsule that surrounds the cholesterol and carries it throughout your bloodstream. The high-density cholesterol is beneficial because its protein capsule carries the cholesterol to the liver, where the cholesterol passes out of your body. The protein capsule surrounding low-density cholesterol, however, carries the cholesterol to your arteries, where it can form plaques that increase the risk of a heart attack or a stroke.

When you exercise, the beneficial high-density cholesterol increases, and the harmful low-density cholesterol decreases. Medical researchers do not yet know why this happens. However, researchers do know that the more exercise you do, the more high-density cholesterol your body produces.

Note that you can raise your high-density cholesterol levels in only two other ways: by taking female hormones and by drinking alcohol. But taking female hormones will make a man impotent, and drinking alcohol does not raise the HDL subfraction that helps to prevent heart attacks.

IT HELPS YOU STAY AWAKE DURING THE DAY

Q *I've been feeling very sleepy in midmorning and midafternoon, even though I get a good night's sleep and am a healthy person. How can I overcome this problem?*

A Midmorning and midafternoon slumps commonly occur if your blood-sugar level is low or the blood circulation to your brain is poor. Of course, the best treatment for tiredness is sleep. A nap of as little as 15 minutes can refresh you for the rest of the day.

Have you been skipping meals? If so, that could be the source of your problem. Going without breakfast, for example, will cause your blood sugar to drop in the morning. Your bloodstream carries only enough sugar to fuel your body for about three minutes. To keep your blood-sugar level from dropping, your liver constantly releases its stored sugar into your bloodstream. However, your liver contains only enough sugar to last about 12 hours. If you skip breakfast, your liver may run out of its stored sugar and your blood sugar will then drop.

Your brain gets most of its energy from sugar supplied by your bloodstream. If your sugar supply is low, your brain may not get enough fuel, which causes you to feel sleepy. You may need to eat regularly to prevent this from happening.

Exercise when you feel sluggish. Jog in place for a few minutes. Stretch your legs out in front of you while you sit in a chair and alternately contract and relax your leg muscles for a few minutes. Stand and stretch by clasping your hands together and reaching your arms up as high as you can. Hold the stretch for 10 seconds; relax. Repeat the arm-stretch routine for a few minutes.

Simple exercises like these will increase your body temperature and make your heart pump more blood through your body, carrying more fuel (sugar) and oxygen to your brain. As a result, you'll feel more alert.

Most people with your problem do not have a serious medical condition. Nevertheless, if the above procedures don't help you, check with your doctor. In some people, sluggishness can be the result of a chronic infection, liver problems, or other medical conditions.

IT HELPS YOU CONCENTRATE

You may believe that when you exercise to the point of

exhaustion you become too tired to think. But, when you exercise, it's your body that becomes tired, not your mind. No matter how much you exercise, you should be able to think and reason at least as clearly as you could before you exercised.

Several studies demonstrate this fact. In one study, several runners were given the same series of standard psychological tests before they exercised and a few hours after they finished competing in a marathon. Each one had exercised nearly to the point of exhaustion—their average weight loss was more than six pounds, their pulse rates were more than 10 beats a minute faster than usual, and they had an average rise in body temperature of more than 2°C.

The test results showed that while the runners were in this semi-exhausted state, they were still able to follow instructions, memorize, perform certain physical tasks, and answer questions as well as they could before they started exercising. In fact, the runners made fewer mistakes on the tests after the marathon.

What this study proves is that people can be alert enough after exercising vigorously to do things such as drive a car or concentrate on a difficult problem at work. The conclusions can also apply to schoolchildren, who should be able to study in class after having exercised vigorously.

While rigorous exercise won't interfere with your concentration, regular exercise will enhance it. As you may have observed from your own experience, after sitting in a classroom or lecture hall for several hours your ability to concentrate and learn gradually deteriorates. And, at work your ability to concentrate usually wanes after lunch.

Studies sponsored by several major corporations found that, without exercise, workers were less productive after lunch, while those who exercised before coming back to work were much more productive. That's why companies such as Xerox and Johnson & Johnson encourage employees to exercise during lunch using company-supplied swimming pools, tracks, and tennis courts.

If you exercise either between classes or during your lunch hour at work, you probably will be as alert as you were at the start of the day.

BUT IT DOESN'T PREVENT COLDS

Q *Since I started running, I haven't had a single cold. I told my doctor about this, and he laughed at me. Can exercise improve your immunity?*

A There is no evidence that exercise protects you from infection. As far as we know, *antibodies* (substances that kill germs) are not affected by exercise.

Yet, I hear many patients say that, like you, they haven't been sick since they started regular exercise. Researchers are studying one possible explanation.

Germs that cause infections in humans usually grow best at 98.6°F, your normal body temperature. Higher temperatures inhibit germs from growing. This is evident in the laboratory. When doctors do a culture test, they put culture samples in a tube, which is placed in an incubator set at exactly 98.6°F. If the temperature in the incubator rises, the germs often don't grow.

When you exercise, your body temperature rises not only during the exercise period, but for four to six hours after you finish exercising. It is possible that because of this rise in body temperature, exercise improves your body's defense system. Nevertheless, this is still just a theory.

2
HOW DO I START OUT?

THE GENETICS OF BEING A GOOD ATHLETE

Certain inherited physical characteristics such as height, weight, body type, and muscle composition can tell scientists a lot about a person's athletic capabilities—whether, for example, a person has the potential to become a great distance runner or would be a better sprinter. Muscle composition is a major factor in determining whether you are better at running longer distances or at sprinting.

Your muscles are made up of two major types of fibers: red, slow-twitch fibers used primarily for endurance and white, fast-twitch ones used primarily for speed and strength. Most people have an equal number of slow- and fast-twitch fibers in their thigh muscles, the muscles that give you power during distance events.

Most successful competitors in 10-kilometer races and marathons however, have a higher proportion of slow-twitch fibers in their thigh muscles—more than 75 percent. And, athletes who compete in shorter, high-intensity speed events such as sprints and 100-yard, 200-yard, and 400-yard events have a higher proportion of white, fast-twitch fibers.

You can find out the ratio of slow-twitch to fast-twitch fibers in your muscles by having a doctor perform a *muscle biopsy*, in which a tiny piece of muscle is cut out and examined under a microscope. This can provide you with interesting and helpful information.

But a muscle biopsy can't tell you everything. A great athlete must have motivation and the ability to handle a tough work load. The most advanced scientific methods can neither determine if you have these important factors nor give them to you.

THE HARD-EASY PRINCIPLE

Q *I read so much about the joy of being fit that I started a jogging program on my 40th birthday. I knew that great athletes train almost every day, so I decided to run every day. The third week into my program, I tore a hamstring muscle and haven't done any exercising since. I think I was injured because my body has a weakness so that I am more likely than others to become injured. Now, I'm afraid to exercise. Can you help me?*

A Many people mistakenly feel that fitness requires a great deal of time. They exercise too much and quickly become injured. Then, they can't exercise at all.

Q *How much exercise do I need to be fit?*

A You need to exercise only for 30 minutes, three times a week. For many of us, exercising more often than that increases our chances of injuring ourselves.

THE 48-HOUR RECOVERY RULE

Q *How much time must I take off between exercise sessions?*

A Every time that you exercise, your muscles are injured. Your muscles are made up of thousands of stringy fibers. Biopsies of skeletal muscles on the day after vigorous exercise show that there is bleeding into the muscle fibers and disruption of their structures.

It takes at least 48 hours for your muscles to heal from exercise. So, most of us would be better off exercising every other day, rather than every day.

Q *But don't champion swimmers and runners exercise at least twice a day? Don't the double workouts help to make them better athletes?*

A Sure, they improve by doing more work, but you should realize that they usually allow 48 hours for their muscles to recover.

Champion marathon runners may run at a four-minute mile pace on their hard days. The next three workouts, however, are usually run at a much slower pace, such as five to eight minutes per mile. Athletes working out twice a day usually follow each hard workout with three easy ones.

During exercise, your muscles and tendons act like rubber bands. They stretch and contract continuously with each movement. As you grow older, however, your muscles and tendons lose much of their elasticity and are more likely to tear.

As a general rule, most people under the age of 35 can use the hard-easy principle in the same sport and remain relatively injury free. Most people over 35 are probably better off exercising every other day, or, if they want to exercise daily, they should alternate sports that stress different parts of their bodies.

Running primarily stresses the muscles in your lower leg; riding a bicycle, the muscles in your upper leg. So, if you alternated running and cycling, you would follow the 48-hour recovery rule. When you run, you allow the upper leg muscles to recover. When you pedal, you allow the lower leg muscles to recover.

If you are more than 60 years of age, you are probably better off exercising only every other day. Your muscles have lost so much elasticity that they recover best if you don't exercise at all on your easy days.

You've learned that fitness requires that you exercise vigorously enough to increase your pulse rate. It doesn't make any difference to your heart which sport you do. This is a universal rule of exercise.

There are other universal rules. You start all sports the same way.

- Every other day, exercise until your muscles feel heavy or hurt and then stop.
- As you round into better shape, you will be able to exercise longer.
- For fitness, you do not need to exercise for more than 30 minutes, three times a week.
- If you want to do more, you can increase the intensity, duration, or frequency of exercise. I recommend that you

start out slowly. Then increase the pace according to how you feel. Slow down when you feel any discomfort and then pick up the pace again as you recover.

WHAT IS THE BEST TIME TO EXERCISE?

Q *My company recently installed an employee exercise center in its headquarters. Do you think it is better to work out before work, at lunchtime, or after work?*

A The best time to exercise is just before you want to do your best work.

After a vigorous workout, you are more alert and better able to concentrate because your circulation and metabolism are stimulated. Your temperature is elevated, your pulse rate is higher than normal, and you continue to burn extra calories.

However, the increased concentration that comes from exercise only lasts four to six hours. Thus, if you exercise early in the morning, you will probably run out of steam around noon and your energy will flag in the afternoon.

HOW TO COMPARE DIFFERENT SPORTS

Q *Which form of exercise requires the most energy: jogging, bicycling, jumping rope, or swimming?*

A The only way you can compare the energy used in different sports is to use common measures, such as the number of calories burned, the amount of oxygen used, or the heartbeat rate achieved. Ten minutes of jumping rope, for example, uses the same amount of energy as 10 minutes of jogging—both make the heart rate quicken to 120 beats a minute.

Jumping rope is commonly believed to take more energy than jogging because most people have to spin a rope at least 80 times a minute to keep it from tangling. Jumping 80 times a minute is hard work and equals running a mile in 7½ minutes, a fairly rapid pace for any noncompetitive runner.

If you exercise two or three times a week and are not training for competition, you will use the same amount of energy jogging a mile, bicycling four miles, or swimming a quarter-mile.

WARMING UP

Q *What is the purpose of a warm-up and how does it improve athletic performance?*

A Every time you work out or play a sport you should start with a few minutes of warm-up activity to prevent muscle injuries, increase the flow of blood to your heart, and help you perform better and enjoy your exercise more.

Muscles are like putty. The temperature of a cold, resting muscle is 98°F. Cold muscles are stiff and are more likely to tear when you exercise them vigorously. If you take time to warm them up to 101°F or 102°F before you work out, your muscles will be soft, pliable, and much more resistant to injury.

Think of your warm-up as a rehearsal for the main sports event. The most effective warm-up activity is one that mimics your sport. For example, runners can warm up by jogging slowly or running in place for about 10 minutes. Figure skaters or hockey players can skate slowly around the rink several times. Tennis players can rally for 10 minutes before a match. Swimmers can swim a few easy laps before a race.

Q *How long does it take to warm up?*

A Five to 10 minutes are all you need. When you start to perspire, your muscles are warmed up—your muscle temperature is higher, more blood is flowing to your heart, and your brain and nervous system are prepared so your muscles will be better coordinated. You will be able to run faster, jump higher, throw farther, swim longer, or lift heavier weights.

Muscle temperature returns to resting level within 45 minutes, so you should schedule your warm-up no more than 45 minutes before your main sports activity.

Q *Does applying heat to your legs before you run help you to exercise better?*

A No. Heating your muscles in a whirlpool bath, with hot packs, or under an infrared lamp just before you run does warm up the muscles. Nevertheless, it does not increase their circulation, which is vital to an improved performance.

Warming up by exercising, though, improves circulation

and raises muscle temperatures one to three degrees. This often results in an ability to jump farther, lift heavier weights, or run faster for a short distance. It also decreases the chances of your developing an irregular heartbeat. Yet, it does not increase endurance, which is necessary for participation in long-term sports, such as marathon races.

Endurance depends on the amount of sugar that is stored in your muscles. If this sugar runs out during exercise, your muscles will begin to ache and you will have difficulty coordinating and contracting them.

Increasing the temperature of your muscles uses up the sugar stored in them at a rapid rate and causes you to tire faster than usual, thereby reducing your endurance.

STRETCHING

Q *Why is it so important to stretch before exercising, and what is the best way to do it?*

A Stretching increases your flexibility by lengthening muscles that have been shortened by exercise. When you exercise muscles they are slightly injured. Then, during the healing process, they shorten. Unless you lengthen them by stretching, tight muscles are more likely to be torn and injured.

You need to stretch those muscles you use most in your chosen sport. A runner or walker needs to stretch the calf and hamstring muscles. A swimmer should concentrate on stretching various arm muscles.

Before you stretch, you must warm up your muscles by exercising them gently and slowly for a few minutes to avoid injury. Never stretch a cold muscle. Stretching itself does not warm up a muscle. The normal temperature of a resting muscle is 98°F. When you exercise a muscle for a few minutes, its temperature goes up to around 102°F. This makes the muscle more pliable and less likely to tear.

Stretch slowly. Stretching too rapidly causes your muscles to contract. When your muscles contract while you're trying to stretch them, their fibers are more prone to tear. Don't go any further than you can reach without strain. Hold for a count of 10 and then relax and repeat the stretch 10 times. Don't bounce or jerk as you stretch.

COOLING DOWN

Q *Can you explain the principle of cooling down and how it can help me after I exercise?*

A Cooling down after exercise that uses your leg muscles can help you avoid some unpleasant aftereffects, including fainting.

Cooling down means to continue exercising at a very slow pace for about five minutes after a vigorous workout. A runner can cool down, for example, by running slowly. Running, or other hard exercise that uses the legs, makes those muscles alternately relax and contract. When the leg muscles relax, the nearby veins expand and fill with blood. When the muscles contract, they push on those veins, squeezing additional blood up to your heart. This action, because the leg muscles are so large, works like a second heart to pump blood through your body.

If you are running or biking hard and then suddenly stop, for instance, your leg muscles stop contracting. Gravity causes the blood to pool in your legs, so not enough may be pumped back up to your brain. You may feel dizzy and pass out. When you take just a few minutes to cool down, however, you gradually ease the pumping action of the leg muscles and avoid dizziness or fainting.

Q *Can a cool-down period prevent muscle soreness?*

A Sportsmedicine experts no longer believe that it can. During vigorous exercise, your body needs a lot of oxygen. Even though you breathe as hard as you can, you may not get all the oxygen you need. That can cause lactic acid (a breakdown product of metabolism) to collect in your bloodstream. We once believed that this buildup of lactic acid causes the muscle soreness many people feel the day after a workout. We now know it doesn't.

Scientists believe that next-day soreness stems from torn muscle fiber caused by exercise.

So, although cooling down can keep you from feeling dizzy and does help clear lactic acid from your bloodstream at a faster rate, it doesn't help you fight day-after aches and pains.

PROPER BREATHING

Q *I have heard that you should breathe exclusively through your nose because it is superior to your mouth in warming air and filtering pollution. Is this true?*

A Exercise greatly increases your body's demand for oxygen. Unfortunately, your nose is simply not big enough to take in enough oxygen during exercise. Also, breathing through your mouth presents no danger.

The amount of air you take in depends largely on the size of the opening through which the air passes on its way to your lungs. The opening at the back of your mouth is about two inches in diameter. The apertures in your nose total less than one-tenth that size.

Nevertheless, when you are at rest, the nose is the breathing apparatus of choice. It can easily admit enough air to satisfy the body's normal oxygen needs and has special equipment to improve air quality. The nose is lined with ridges called *turbinates* that heat incoming air and with tiny hairs that help filter out pollutants.

The mouth lacks these special warming and filtering features, but you need not worry about damaging your lungs by breathing through your mouth while exercising in cold weather or in polluted air.

Air taken in through the mouth is warmed by the blood under the surface lining of your bronchial tubes that lead to and from your lungs. Air taken in at minus 40°F will be warmed by more than 100 degrees before it reaches your lungs, which is more than adequate to protect your lungs from damage.

Q *Can air pollution cause damage when I exercise?*

A As for pollutants, those inhaled though the mouth during exercise normally are cleared quickly and efficiently by your lungs. The bronchial tubes are lined with small mucous glands and tiny hairs, or *cilia*. These work in tandem: the mucus traps pollutants. The constantly waving cilia sweep the mucus with the trapped pollutants back into your mouth, where they are swallowed with your saliva and eventually excreted. Lungs not damaged by smoking or disease are easily able to clear your body of up to two tons of pollutants a year.

EXERCISE PROGRAMS AND FITNESS CLUBS

Q *I would like to exercise, but each time I start an exercise program, I drop out. Would I be better off in a formal program?*

A Surprise! People involved in organized programs tend to stop exercising more often than people who work out on their own. A study conducted at the University of Wisconsin at Madison shows that the drop-out rate for supervised exercise enthusiasts was 45 percent, while 30 percent of those who went it alone failed to continue their own program.

The Wisconsin researchers contend that lack of time is the most frequent reason for dropping out of a group exercise program. It takes time to pack your gym bag and travel to and from an exercise group. And, you have to work out when and where the group gathers. You may be able to save time by exercising at home according to your own schedule.

Whichever you prefer—group or solo exercise—make sure the program realistically fits your needs. The stress and strain of trying to get across town for an after-work exercise class may be more trouble than it's worth. If you can find a convenient, supervised program, by all means join. A program conducted at your place of work during lunch break or right after work would be ideal.

Q *I am forced to follow an irregular schedule by the demands of my job. What is the best way to schedule time? Are there any supervised programs for people like me?*

A You might be better off with an exercise regimen that you can follow on your own and vary to meet your needs. For example, if you are a runner who travels a lot on business, you can jog in place in your hotel room. If you work all day and get home late, you could jog on a small trampoline set up in your bedroom. Stationary bicycles are good for people with unpredictable schedules. You can ride a stationary bike any time and in any weather.

If your schedule forces you to miss a few exercise classes or home workouts, don't despair. The remedy depends on how long you go without exercise. Once you stop working out, the endurance that is so vital to fitness disappears quickly. You can lose your stamina in only two weeks. If this happens to you, go back to the beginning and work up to your former level of exercise. If you did it before, you can do it again.

Q *Fitness clubs are springing up all over the country. Some will make you happy and fit; others will make you sad and poor. How can you tell the good clubs from the bad?*

A Check the exercise equipment and the people who run the club. Ideally, you should find two kinds of equipment and facilities: those that will make your heart and lungs strong and those that will strengthen your muscles.

For heart and lung fitness, you can ride a stationary bicycle, jog on a treadmill or track, attend aerobic dance classes, swim, play racquetball, jump rope or jump on a small trampoline, or use rowing or skiing machines.

For muscle strength you can push on special strength-training machines or lift weights.

Stay away from clubs that promote gimmicky equipment and claim it will do the work for you. Riding a bicycle with motor-driven pedals or being shaken by a vibrating machine will not make you fit.

Visit the club at the time when you expect to use it. A club that is not crowded at 10 A.M. may be packed at noon or right after work. If there are large crowds, you must wait to use equipment, you won't have much room on the aerobic dance floor, and the staff won't have much time to give you individual attention.

Make sure the instructors have undergone special training to teach you to exercise correctly. Beware of clubs where the staff is selling, not instructing. If they are more interested in selling you food supplements than teaching you how to exercise, look elsewhere. You become fit by exercising, not by eating. Besides, you can get all the nutrients you need by eating a well-balanced diet.

According to the Federal Trade Commission, most complaints about fitness clubs concern high-pressure sales methods, exaggerated promises about facilities, and clubs that take your money and then suddenly close.

Ask questions. Make sure you understand what you are getting for your money before you commit yourself to a program. And, let your better business bureau know if the club doesn't live up to its promises.

ENDURANCE: HOW DO MEN AND WOMEN COMPARE?

Q *Is it true that women have greater endurance than men?*

A Possibly! Women have more stored energy than men because they have a higher percentage of body fat. They also have less weight to carry because their bones and muscles are lighter. That counts if you're on a cross-country skiing trip and get lost or if you plan to swim the English Channel. In these cases, a woman will be more likely to endure. For most sports, however, strength and speed are more important than endurance.

There are many examples of great feats of endurance by women. For instance, Canada's Cindy Nichols holds the world record for swimming the English Channel round-trip, which she did nonstop in 20 hours. That's more than ten hours faster than the best time achieved by a man. Another example is England's Wendy Brooks, who holds the France-to-England swimming record, which is more than 40 minutes faster than the record held by a man for the same distance.

The average fit woman can endure longer, in part, because she is 25 percent fat, compared to the average fit male who is 15 percent fat. And fat provides the most efficient storage of body fuel.

Q *How do the muscles draw energy from the food that I eat?*

AMuscles can use carbohydrates, fats, and proteins for energy. Carbohydrates are the chief fuel for intense exercise because, unlike fats, they can be used without oxygen. Fats are the most-used body fuel because so much can be stored. One pound of stored fat in fat cells contains 3,500 calories. Carbohydrates can be stored only as glycogen in the liver and muscles. Each gram of glycogen requires three additional grams of water so that one pound of stored liver or muscle glycogen contains only 250 calories or one-fourteenth as much as for the same weight as fat. Proteins are a minor source of energy for exercise, for the body has no way to store extra protein.

SECOND WIND

Q*I have often gotten a burst of energy in the middle of exercise. It sometimes occurs when I am out for a run, or while I've been playing a hard, fast-moving game of basket-ball with friends. I become very short of breath and tired and feel ready to quit. But suddenly I feel a wave of energy come over me and am ready for more. Is that a "second wind"? Is there really such a thing?*

AWhen you become short of breath during exercise and feel so tired that you want to give up, there is only one way you are going to recover: slow down so your body gets the oxygen it needs.

During sustained exercise, your body requires considerable amounts of oxygen. The harder you work out, the more oxygen you need. Sometimes you exercise so intensely that your heart is unable to pump all the oxygen-rich blood your muscles need, which can cause an oxygen deficit. When this happens, your muscles become tired and feel heavy. You may lose control over your muscles and feel cramps in them. You will also breathe hard and pant as your body tries to take in more air.

To compensate for this oxygen deficit, your body naturally slows down. But, you won't feel it because you're still working equally hard just to help your body catch up. Because you aren't exercising as intensely as before, your body requires less oxygen, and you gradually are able to fill your need for oxygen. When you no longer have an oxygen deficit, your muscles will hurt less and you'll feel less tired and more refreshed. That's when you pick up your pace. Again, you won't notice the change in pace, just the renewed vigor.

So, yes, there is such a thing as a "second wind." Only now you know it isn't magical, but simply a natural way for your body to regroup so you can exercise longer.

EXTRA WEIGHT AND THE COMPETITIVE EDGE

Q *I know that extra weight can tire you, but just how important is extra fat when you walk, run, or ride a bicycle?*

A For every extra pound you gain, your muscles will require more oxygen, which will make your heart beat faster when exercising. The effect movement has on your heartbeat is based on the following formula: work equals force times distance. Obviously, the more force that is exerted, the more work you have to do. During slow walking, your heart will beat one more time per minute for every 2 pounds of additional fat, and your lungs will take in one more pint of air. So, if you are 20 pounds overweight, during walking your heart will beat 10 times more per minute and you will take in 20 more pints of air. Those 20 extra pounds will slow you down one to two minutes for every mile you walk.

During rigorous exercise, the figures become more significant. Ten extra pounds of fat will slow a runner more than 20 minutes during a marathon. The same rule applies to riding a bicycle.

Q *Will lighter shoes help me lower my race times?*

A Runners often wear such light shoes that their feet are not supported properly. Or, they wear shirts with holes in them or even tear some of the paper off their numbers in an attempt to shed a few extra ounces to gain speed.

Bicycle racers try to do the same thing by drilling holes in the chains of their bikes. Drilling 30 holes in a chain wheel will make a bicycle one-half ounce lighter. This loss in weight will allow the racer to go three yards faster in one hour while climbing a hill with a 10 percent grade. That's a lot of effort for negligible results. If the racer lost two pounds of body fat, he or she could go 200 yards ahead with the same amount of effort.

3
HOW CAN I MAKE MY HEART STRONGER?

CARDIOVASCULAR FITNESS

Q *What is cardiovascular fitness and how can I attain it?*

A The following is a handy general formula for achieving cardiovascular fitness:

100 beats a minute
for 30 minutes
three times a week

Fitness refers to your heart. Most exercise physiologists recommend that, for fitness, you try to exercise vigorously enough to raise your pulse rate to at least 100 beats a minute for 30 minutes, three times a week. (More on this formula below.)

Q *How can I strengthen my heart?*

A Your heart is a muscle. To strengthen any muscle, you must exercise it against resistance.

Here's how you make your heart work against extra resistance. When you exercise, you contract and relax your skeletal muscles. When you relax your muscles, they allow the veins near them to fill up with blood. When you contract your muscles, they push against the veins near them and squeeze the blood from the veins toward your heart. This causes extra blood to return to your heart.

Your heart is a muscular balloon. It fills up with blood and then squeezes the blood from its chambers to your body. The more blood that returns to the heart, the greater the force that the heart must exert to pump blood through your body. The extra blood that is pumped to your heart during exercise is what makes your heart stronger.

We can tell how much extra blood is returning to your heart by measuring your pulse. Studies show that you must increase your pulse rate at least 20 beats a minute above resting to make it stronger. That comes out to around 100 beats a minute.

Q *I have heard that you must increase your heart rate to 60 percent of its maximum to improve cardiovascular fitness. What does this mean?*

A There are purists among you who will not be satisfied with the explanation of 100 beats a minute. You know there is a formula that says to train your heart you must exercise vigorously enough to raise your pulse rate to 60 percent of its maximum.

The maximum pulse rate is the fastest that your heart can beat and still pump blood through your body. It works out to about 220 minus your age.

MAXIMUM PULSE RATE FOR YOUR AGE GROUP

Maximum Pulse Rate	Age
210	10
200	20
190	30
180	40
170	50
160	60
150	70
140	80

Sixty percent of your maximum pulse rate comes out somewhere between 100 and 120, but the numbers aren't exact enough to make 100 beats a minute incorrect as the minimal training pulse rate.

Q *Is 10 minutes of exercise three times a week sufficient?*

A You can develop a strong heart on just 10 minutes of continuous exercise, but 30 minutes will make it even stronger. You will receive diminishing returns per time spent when you exercise much longer than 30 minutes.

You cannot be fit on one workout a week. You can be fit on

two, but three will be even better. As I mentioned earlier, exercising vigorously every day increases the chance of injuring yourself. Most people are better off exercising every other day, so three workouts a week are best for most people.

HOW TO TAKE YOUR EXERCISE PULSE

Unless you raise the rate of your heartbeat to at least 100 beats per minute, you can't really strengthen your heart by exercising. You can gauge your heartbeat by taking your exercise pulse.

Q *How do I take my exercise pulse?*

A The best time to take your exercise pulse is immediately after a workout session. The best place to measure this pulse is, for men, beside their Adam's apple, and for women, the spot where the Adam's apple would be. The strongest pulses are in the neck and in the groin; the neck pulses are easier to feel because they are close to the surface.

To take your pulse, put your index finger on the side of your neck where you feel the beat. Count the beats for six seconds. Multiply that number by 10 to get your pulse rate per minute. Because the pulse rate slows down very quickly after you stop exercising, you must not count for more than six seconds. If you do, you will receive a falsely low count.

Be aware, however, that the carotid body nerve sensors in the neck's blood vessels are hypersensitive to pressure. Some especially sensitive people can experience a drop in blood pressure or a slowing of their heart rates if they exert pressure on these vessels.

(Wearing a tight collar can also irritate these nerves and cause faintness. If a collar presses too hard against the carotid body, which controls the heart rate, the amount of blood pumped to the brain may drop, causing temporary dizziness.)

The most common method of taking a pulse is to put your fingers on your wrist. Often, the wrist pulse is difficult to measure because the blood vessels in the wrist are small and do not transmit a strong beat to the fingertips. Nurses and doctors use this method to avoid scaring the patient by reaching for his or her neck.

Putting your hand over your heart is not an efficient measure, either. The heart is separated from your fingers by the thick chest wall, so your ability to feel each beat is restricted.

USING BREATHING TO MEASURE YOUR EXERCISE PULSE

Q *Taking my pulse during exercise is very distracting. Is there any other way I can tell how fast my heart is beating?*

A You never have to take your pulse during exercise. You can tell how fast your heart is beating by paying close attention to how you breathe.

Two heart rates should concern you when you exercise. The first is the minimal heart rate that strengthens your heart to make you fit. The second is the maximal heart rate that is the fastest your heart can beat and still pump blood through your body.

To strengthen your heart, you must increase your heart rate at least 20 beats a minute beyond your resting heart rate. That will be your minimal heart-training rate. You can easily tell when you have reached your minimal rate because, at that point, your body will require more oxygen than it does at rest.

You will start breathing more deeply and rapidly, but will feel comfortable and will still be able to talk.

When exercising at your maximal heart rate, you will gasp for breath and will not be able to talk.

For fitness, you should work up to the point where you can exercise continuously for 20 to 30 minutes, three times a week, at your minimal heart rate. You should just begin to increase the depth of your breathing, but you should not become short of breath. Some people who exercise at their maximal heart rate develop irregular heart beats. Their hearts may stop pumping blood through their bodies and they may pass out.

HOW TO TELL IF YOUR HEART IS GETTING STRONGER

Q *What is the surest way to tell if my exercise program is working?*

A A simple way to test the effectiveness of your exercise program is to find out how well it is training your heart. This is done by measuring your *recovery pulse index*: how much your pulse slows down one minute after you stop exercising.

Your pulse rate is proportional to the amount of blood pumped with each heartbeat. Your recovery pulse rate is proportionate to your heart's fitness. The stronger the heart, the more quickly it recovers from exercise and the less frequently it must beat.

A quick recovery signifies a strong heart. It also indicates the well-being of other functions of the body. It indirectly gauges how quickly your body rids itself of the waste products of metabolism, primarily lactic acid. As lactic acid is cleansed from the bloodstream, the pulse rate slackens.

In addition, a rapid recovery indicates the efficiency of the chemicals (located in the muscles) that regulate the use of oxygen and fuel. As muscles become better trained through regular workouts, they require less oxygen and less work on the part of the heart.

Q *I realize that recovery rate is an excellent way to measure my level of fitness. How do I test my recovery rate?*

A To test yourself: Work out as hard as you can for five minutes. Be careful. If you have a weak heart, this can be dangerous. When you stop, immediately place one or two fingers on either side of your neck where you will feel a strong pulse.

Count the pulse for six seconds. Then multiply that number by 10. This gives you your pulse rate per minute. It is important to count only for six seconds: heartbeat rate decreases very quickly once you cease exercising. If you count your pulse for longer than six seconds you will get an incorrectly low reading.

Exactly one minute after you have stopped exercising, take your pulse in the same way for six seconds. Multiply by 10 once more.

Now deduct the second figure from the first. If the second count is not at least 30 beats less than the first, you are not in good shape.

WILL EXERCISE CAUSE A HEART ATTACK?

Q *I've been thinking of starting an exercise program, but I've heard of people doing so, and then suddenly dropping* *dead. How can I know whether regular exercise will hurt me? I am a 51-year-old man.*

A First, check with your physician. However, the chance of a man dying during exercise is estimated to be one in 5 million; for a woman, it is one in 17 million.

You can never be absolutely certain in medicine, but research—and much has been done on this subject—indicates that you should be careful about exercise if you have a strong family history of heart attacks, strokes, hardening of the arteries, or diabetes; if you smoke, have high blood pressure, or a high blood-fat level; if you experience chest pain, particularly when you exercise; if mild exercise makes you short of breath; or if your resting heart rate is higher than 80 beats a minute.

If you have any of these symptoms, your physician may want to conduct tests to find out if exercise is likely to harm you.

SHOULD I GET AN EXERCISE EKG?

Q *I am 35 years old and would like to start an exercise program. Should I get an exercise electrocardiogram before I begin?*

A An *exercise electrocardiogram*, in which a patient is monitored while exercising at increasing speeds, lets your physician and you know how much exercise your heart can tolerate. If you are generally healthy, it isn't necessary to take an exercise electrocardiogram before you begin an exercise program.

Nevertheless, taking an exercise electocardiogram is recommended if you have any heart-risk factors such as high blood pressure, a high blood-fat level, irregular heartbeats, unexplained dizziness, or a family history of heart disease, or if you smoke.

An exercise electrocardiogram is not a definitive procedure. If any abnormalities show up, you will have to take further tests. The procedure itself is very safe, with a less than one in 20,000 chance of causing a heart attack.

WARNING SIGNS

Q *My father died of a heart attack, and I am terrified of dying during exercise. How can you tell that your heart can't function properly when you exercise?*

A Your heart will provide warning signs if you are overtaxing it. Everyone, especially the novice exerciser and anyone over 40, should be alert for these signals during and after a workout:

- chest pain
- nausea or dizziness
- shortness of breath persisting five minutes after the workout
- a pulse rate that remains elevated at 110 beats per minute or higher for 15 minutes or longer after you stop exercising.

All of these symptoms have to do with the increased oxygen demands that vigorous exercise puts on your body. In a vigorous workout, your muscles require large amounts of oxygen, while the ordinary oxygen demands of the rest of your body remain undiminished. Extra oxygen must be delivered by your blood, which must be pumped at a harder and faster than normal rate.

Chest pain during exercise may indicate a partially blocked blood supply to the heart itself. Any blockage or narrowing of the coronary arteries that bring blood to the heart's surface (virtually the heart's only oxygen supply) is likely to make itself felt during exercise, when the rest of your muscles need so much oxygen. If the heart muscle is being deprived of oxygen, it will signal the fact in the form of chest pain.

Nausea or dizziness during exercise may be signs of a weak heart or an irregular heartbeat. If your heart is not strong enough to accommodate the demands of exercise, it may not be able to supply your brain with a constant and adequate oxygen supply. Similarly, a missed heartbeat may temporarily deprive the brain of oxygen. In either case, you may become nauseated or dizzy, or you may even faint.

Q *Often when I exercise vigorously I have a difficult time getting my breathing back to normal, even half an hour after jogging. Is this dangerous? Do I have a weak heart?*

A It is normal to breathe harder than usual when you exercise. This is part of the body's mechanism for supplying increased oxygen. But, you should be able to catch up on your oxygen needs and breathe normally within a few seconds after your workout ends. If you are still short of breath about five minutes after you stop exercising, it may be because your heart is not strong enough for the extra stress you're putting on it.

By the same token, a pulse elevated to 120 to 160 beats a minute by exercise should drop to below 110 beats a minute within 15 minutes after you stop exercising. If it fails to do this, your heart may be protesting against demands it is not strong enough to meet.

If you experience any of the warning signals, take no chances. Persisting in hard exercise when you feel any of these symptoms means you are courting a possible heart attack or stroke. Suspend your exercise program immediately and see your physician.

Your doctor may recommend an exercise electrocardiogram, or *stress test*, which monitors your heart while you exercise. Though not foolproof, a stress test can help to diagnose cases of abnormalities of the heart.

COLD SHOWERS

Q *After I work out, I enjoy a cold shower. Can cold showers be dangerous?*

A Most people can safely take a cold shower, but it can be dangerous if you have high blood pressure, a weak heart, or if you have been drinking alcohol.

When skin comes in contact with cold water, the body tries to conserve heat by narrowing blood vessels near the skin's surface. Since the same amount of blood is contained in a smaller area, the blood pressure will rise. The heart will have to work much harder to pump blood against the increased pressure.

If you already suffer from high blood pressure, very cold water on your skin can drive your pressure high enough to burst blood vessels and cause a stroke.

A healthy heart should be able to continue to beat regularly and pump blood against the increased pressure. A weak heart, however, may not have enough power to handle the increased resistance and it may start to beat irregularly.

Drinking alcohol before taking a cold shower also can lead to irregular heartbeats. Skin contact with cold water can result in *hypothermia*, which is lower-than-normal body temperature. Normally, your body will respond by shivering—a process that helps it to produce sufficient heat to maintain body temperature. But, alcohol raises the shiver response threshold; it takes a lower body temperature to trigger this rapid contraction and relaxation of the muscles. As a result, your body temperature may remain low, increasing the risks of hypothermia and irregular heartbeats.

PART II

4

AN A-TO-Z OF QUESTIONS AND ANSWERS ABOUT CARDIOVASCULAR FITNESS AND SPORTS

Everyone wants to be fit, but many people don't know what fitness means. To attain cardiovascular fitness, you must strengthen your heart muscle, and this requires continuous exercise at a reasonably brisk level. It is difficult for most people to become fit by playing tennis, for instance, since few tennis players have enough skill to keep the ball going long enough to strengthen their heart muscles. If you think your calisthenics are making you fit, you're almost assuredly kidding yourself. Calisthenics are rarely done vigorously enough or continuously enough for heart improvement.

This section includes some important descriptive information about the sports that usually promote cardiovascular fitness, as well as a representative collection of questions asked about this subject. It is by no means intended to serve as a comprehensive text on the topic. I hope this chapter will answer many of your questions and inspire you to become fit.

AEROBIC DANCE

Aerobic dancing is sweeping the country, and well it should. It's more than just fun. It can be a ticket to fitness. It can be every bit as effective in strengthening your heart as running, cycling, or swimming. It's a natural for women who like to move to a beat. And, lots of men who aren't interested in exercising in other sports are interested in dancing. Aerobic dancing can make them fit.

In aerobic dancing, an instructor leads you through an exercise program set to music. When you exercise, you should warm up, stretch, train your heart, and then cool down. This same sequence of events is built into every aerobic dance program.

It doesn't matter whether you're in or out of shape. Everyone can dance. However, if you are out of shape, make sure that you start out at your own pace. In the first six weeks, more than 65 percent of all beginners end up with lower leg pains.

Q *I have never been fit before because I hated to exercise. Recently, I discovered aerobic dancing and I love it. Now, I can't dance at all because I have horrible pain on the inside front of my lower leg. My doctor called it a stress fracture. Why did this happen to me and what can I do to heal faster?*

A You were injured because you tried to keep up with people who were in better shape than you. Then, when you felt a pain in your leg telling you that you had an injury, you didn't stop exercising. Most likely, if you had stopped dancing when you first felt pain, you would have missed only a few days.

All exercises that are done on your feet stress primarily the structures in your lower legs. The greater part of the shock of your foot striking the ground is transmitted to your foot and lower leg. Also, after you land on your heel you must raise yourself up on your toes before you can step off to the other foot. When you do this, your calf muscles and Achilles tendons are subjected to greater forces than are exerted on any other muscles and tendons. This great force increases their chance of injury also.

Now, you must wait for a crack on the surface of your bone to heal. This can take from eight weeks to a year, depending on your body's own natural healing powers and your willingness to stop dancing until you can do so without pain.

BASKETBALL

Basketball players, like all athletes, need endurance to excel. But, the kind of stamina required for basketball is not the same as that required for running a marathon, for instance. Running long distances, in fact, could interfere with a hoopster's skills.

Enjoyed by 24 million Americans, basketball is a sport characterized by very fast, continuous forward movement, sudden lateral shifts, and a lot of jumping. During a game, basketball players rarely run more than 20 yards or 30 yards continuously. Long-distance training of five miles or more can actually impair jumping ability.

Muscles are made up of two major types of fiber. Fast-twitch fibers govern speed and strength, while slow-twitch fibers govern endurance. When you spend a lot of time running long, slow distances, you develop slow-twitch endurance fibers at the expense of strength-and-speed fibers. This will help you run for a longer period of time, but it will reduce your ability to run fast and jump high.

Q *How can I improve my athletic skills for basketball, skills such as endurance, speed, and jumping?*

A The best way for a hoopster to improve endurance is simply to play basketball and, perhaps, run fast, short sprints. To be able to jump higher, you need to strengthen and quicken your leg muscles. You can accomplish this by running sprints or doing deep knee-squats with a heavy force on your shoulders, such as a barbell or a special strength-training machine. Run sprints or do the squats two or three times a week.

The key to training for a higher jump is strength training. The stronger you are, the higher you'll jump. Kent Benson, a former all-American at Indiana Univeristy, picked up 13 inches on his vertical jump in just six weeks of strength training.

For effective strength training, you have to use your muscles in the same way that you use them when you jump. Choose the heaviest weight you can, put the weight on your shoulders and then, starting in a squat position, raise and lower your body consecutively eight times. You can also do this exercise on a machine called a *leaper*. If you use the machine, you can do the exercise without supervision. Otherwise, make sure you do it under close supervision, since a wrong move while you are holding a heavy weight can lead to serious injury.

Do this every other day until you can do 12 repetitions. Then you're ready for a heavier weight. Add 5 pounds to 10 pounds and go back to 8 repetitions, gradually working up to 12.

If you want to increase your speed, you should run the same distance you run when you play basketball. The best way to train is to run 10 dashes of 20-yards each as quickly as you can three days a week. Never do this kind of training on consecutive days.

CALISTHENICS

Q *Are calisthenics considered good exercise?*

A If done properly, calisthenics—isolated muscle exercises such as sit-ups, push-ups, and jumping jacks—can be good exercise. However, most people rest so much between each exercise that they don't get the continuous exercise they need to strengthen their hearts.

If you rest between sets of exercises, say from sit-ups to jumping jacks, your pulse rate slows down immediately. That means you have to start all over again to get your pulse rate back up.

Also, isolated muscle exercises tire you more quickly by putting a strain on those muscles. For example, when you do a push-up you're expending the same amount of energy that you do when taking a step, because in both cases you're carrying the same weight, which is your body. But, your arm muscles will tire much more quickly than your legs will, since when you walk you're distributing the force over a great mass. Because you will tire quickly, you probably won't get as much exercise doing push-ups as you would walking.

Q *Will calisthenics help me burn calories and lose weight?*

A Unless you do them for at least 20 minutes without stopping, doing calisthenics won't burn many calories. By concentrating only on individual muscle groups, calisthenics burn fewer than 200 calories per hour. In comparison, rac-quetball can burn 800 calories per hour; disco dancing, 400 calories per hour; and running at the rate of 6 MPH, 600 calories per hour.

Q *Can I become stronger by doing calisthenics such as push-ups?*

A Calisthenics will probably not make your muscles stronger, either. To strengthen muscles you have to exercise against resistance using increasingly heavier weights. By increasing the number of repetitions of an exercise like push-ups, you will increase your endurance, but not your strength.

CYCLING

The more than 44 million American bicyclists include serious competitors who square off on the roads as well as fitness enthusiasts who pedal in front of their television sets. Some want to win races, others want to strengthen their heart muscles, and many want to shed pounds of fat. On the road to success, cyclists may experience injuries, lack of improvement, and other disappointments.

Regardless of which type of cyclist you are, you'll be able to relate to many of the questions in this section, since you probably have shared some of these goals and setbacks too.

Fitting a Bicycle

Before you cycle, make sure your bicycle fits your body. Like an ill-fitting pair of running shoes, a bicycle that fits you poorly can make you uncomfortable and may even injure you.

Q *Can you explain an easy method of choosing the correct size in a bicycle?*

A Begin by choosing the correct frame size. To do this, take off your shoes and stand very straight. Use a yardstick to measure the distance from the ground to the top of your hipbone. Subtract 13¾ inches from that number to get the correct bicycle frame size for your height. For example, if the distance from the ground to your hip is 39 inches, subtract 13¾ inches and get 25¼ inches. That means you need a 25-inch bicycle frame. Most models are available in 19-inch to 25-inch sizes, and some manufacturers also make 27-inch frames that you can order through your local bicycle shop.

Next, adjust the seat properly. A seat set too low can cause knee pain; if set too high, it can cause lower back pain. Set the seat height by moving one pedal to its lowest position. Ask another person to steady the bike while you get on. Then, adjust the height of the seat until the knee of the leg on the lowered pedal is slightly bent when you sit. Then go for a ride. If your pelvis moves up and down as you pedal, the set is too high and should be adjusted. You should sit comfortably in the seat when you pedal.

Now, tilt the seat so the front is slightly higher than the back. The slight tilt will prevent you from sliding forward as you pedal.

Next, adjust the seat either closer to or farther from the handlebars so that when you put the ball of your foot on the pedal your knee will be directly over the center of the pedal. This position helps you use the full power of each pedal stroke.

The way you set the handlebars depends largely on how fast you ride. If you set them low, you will ride in a bent-over position and will encounter less wind resistance; pedaling will be easier so you can go faster. That's why racers set their handlebars so low. If you set them too low, however, you may strain your back. Experiment to find a handlebar position that feels best to you.

Then, go out and enjoy yourself while getting fit.

Bicycle Touring

Q *I have heard that a sport called bicycle touring is a great way to get fit. What is bicycle touring and where can I find out more about it?*

A An increasing number of people are discovering that bicycle touring is a way to get fit while traveling and meeting new people.

There are many organized bicycle tours throughout the world. Some consist of just a few people from your area, others are major rallies with several thousand bicyclers from various parts of the world.

The big bicycle tours are highly organized productions arranged by various bicycling societies. Many of them use college campuses as home base. If you join such a tour, you will sleep in one of the college dorms and eat in the college cafeteria. Since many of the organizations that run these bicycle tours are nonprofit, they offer room and board for a three-day weekend for less than $100.

You will classify yourself according to your bicycling abilty, from Class A to Class D. Class A bicyclers are the most experienced and usually train by bicycling at least 70 miles a week. If you are in this class, you can expect to cover up to

100 miles a day, moving at about 18 MPH. Class B bicyclers cover 60 to 70 miles a day at 12-15 MPH. Class C bicyclers cover 30 to 40 miles a day and ride at about 10 MPH. In this class, tours include a *sweep*, someone who trails along to make sure no one gets lost along the way. Class D bicyclers are the novices, and a touring group for this class is best for a family that includes children. If you fall into this category, you will cover 10 miles to 20 miles a day, ride at about 8 MPH, and make frequent stops—depending on the ability of the majority of the group.

The major bicycle tours also offer evening activities, including lectures on nutrition and health as well as on buying, maintaining, and riding bicycles. For adults, there is often dancing and for children, movies.

If you are interested in learning more about bicycle touring, send one dollar to Bicycle U.S.A., Suite 209, 6707 Whitestone Road, Baltimore, MD 21207.

Bicycling Safety and Comfort

Q *I want to take up cycling on the roads but my family says it's much too dangerous and I could get myself killed. Is this true?*

A For safety, all bicycle riders should wear helmets; for comfort, they should wear gloves and shorts or pants made especially for the sport.

Last year, more than 1,000 bicyclers in the United States died while riding. Seventy-five percent of those who died were hit by cars and of these, more than 90 percent died from head injuries. If your head hits the ground while you're bicycling, it will hit with a force of at least 450 pounds. A helmet absorbs this enormous force by cushioning your head.

Q *What's the best type of helmet for bike riding?*

A Most bicycle racers wear leather helmets, which are lighter than the hard-shelled plastic ones. For most people, I recommend the plastic helmets, which offer more protection and cost about $40. But, any helmet is effective only if it fits tightly. When you try one on, make sure that it does not move after you fasten the chin strap. And, make sure the chin strap is tightly fastened when you ride.

Q *If I do fall how do I protect myself?*

A There is one important rule to follow if you fall: stay on your bicycle. This way, you'll fall on your side; it is much safer to scrape the skin on your leg than to hit your head.

Q *Is there any special clothing or gear I can wear to make a long bike ride more comfortable?*

A What you wear can make a big difference in your bicycling enjoyment. Buy a good pair of bicycling shorts or pants. These prevent uncomfortable binding because they usually are made of double-knit material that stretches as your thigh muscles expand during exercise. Saddle sores—chafing from the bicycle seat—have ruined many a country bicycle ride. To prevent these sores, make sure your shorts or pants have a chamois lining on the crotch area.

It's also a good idea to wear gloves to help prevent blisters, calluses, and abrasions. Gloves designed specifically for bicyclers are usually made of leather with the top constructed of fishnet material to permit ventilation. Since leather stretches, make sure you buy gloves that feel tight when you first try them on.

Q *Recently, I was out on a bicycle ride with my wife when it started to rain. She fell and broke her collarbone. What could we have done to minimize her chance of falling?*

A First, you should have stopped bicycling for a few minutes. The most dangerous time to bicycle is when it first starts to rain. That's when rubber, sand, oil, and stones that are on the road mix with water, making the roads extremely slippery. After a few minutes, these particles are washed away, making it safer to bicycle.

Second, you could have let some of the air out of your tires to widen them. The bicycle becomes more stable as more rubber touches the ground.

Finally, it's important to slow down when the roads become slippery. The more cautious you are, the less chance you have of falling.

Stationary Bicycles

Q *I exercise outdoors regularly by running, cycling, and* *playing tennis. I get frustrated when faced with several rainy days that can make it miserable or even impossible to play sports. Can you recommend an indoor sport to help tide me through these times and not lose my fitness?*

A Riding a stationary bicycle is a good exercise for rain or shine.

You can go up to four days without exercising before you lose much strength or endurance. After that, your muscles start becoming smaller, the levels of chemicals that help your muscles to process oxygen become lower, your heart pumps less blood with each beat, and your overall strength and endurance start to diminish. Riding a stationary bicycle will prevent this deterioration while you wait for better weather.

Many stationary bicycles have such light flywheels that they don't permit smooth pedaling when you increase the resistance against the pedals. The best ones contain a heavy flywheel that is attached by a chain to the main wheel of your pedals.

Q *I want to begin exercising with my new stationary bicycle. What do I need to know before I start? How long can I pedal without becoming sore?*

A Start by pedaling slowly without resistance until your legs feel heavy or hurt, or you feel tired. Then stop and rest a day. Do this until you work up to pedaling steadily for 30 minutes every other day—all you need for fitness.

If you want a more vigorous workout after that, adjust the resistance knob. Start out by riding without resistance. When you feel warmed up, increase the resistance just a little. If you feel tired or your muscles hurt, lessen the resistance. Gradually try to increase the amount of time you spend riding against resistance.

HEAT TREATMENTS

Q *I have heard that heat treatments are an excellent way to treat sore muscles. How do heat treatments differ and which is the best?*

A Heat is used to treat many sports-related injuries. Physicians, trainers, and physical therapists use a variety of heat sources to warm up a muscle to help promote healing of injuries such as pulled hamstrings, runner's knee, or tennis elbow.

An injured muscle can be warmed by exercising it gently or using hot packs, wet towels, a sauna, whirlpool, or infrared heat lamp, as well as ultrasound, shortwave, and microwave machines. Moist towels create the same effect as a hot-water bottle. The choice of dry or moist heat is usually a matter of personal comfort, not effectiveness.

How you deliver the heat does make a difference, however. The rays of an infrared heat lamp will heat the skin before they heat the muscle deep inside your body. On the other hand, an ultrasound machine will heat the muscle without heating the skin. So, an ultrasound machine generates more heat to the muscle than a heat lamp.

All methods of applying heat to an injury can damage muscles and skin and, therefore, must be used with caution. This is especially important to consider if you are selecting and applying your own heat treatment. Heat packs and heat lamps can raise skin temperature five to 10 degrees—enough to injure it.

Q *Is there any danger in heat treatments such as whirlpools?*

A Even whirlpools can damage your skin. They should never be set higher than 113°F. A temperature of 102°F will have the same therapeutic effect as the higher temperature.

Shortwave and microwave applications penetrate the skin about three centimeters below the surface. Ultrasound machines penetrate deepest of all and cause raised tissue temperature within a few seconds. These treatments should be applied only by a professional.

There are several precautions to take when applying heat. Always remove the source of heat if your skin starts to burn or hurt. Never apply heat to an injury until all swelling has stopped—usually about 48 hours after you suffer the injury. Heat can then be used to relax muscle spasms around the injury, dilate your blood vessels, and increase the blood flow to bring increased amounts of vital nutrients to the site to promote healing. Many physicians believe that the heat itself speeds the healing process.

Q *When should I rule out heat treatments completely?*

A While heat is often an effective treatment of injuries, there are times when it should not be applied. Never apply heat to: (1) any injury in which numbness or loss of feeling has occurred; (2) eyes or genitals—areas so sensitive that even a minor increase in temperature may be damaging; and (3) bones that have had metal pins, screws, or plates inserted into them. Heat can cause the metal to expand at a different rate than the bone, which, in turn, can cause the bone to break.

Q *Do analgesic balms help heal a pulled muscle?*

A Analgesic balms contain mostly oil of wintergreen, which is nothing more than concentrated aspirin. They are anesthetics that help alleviate muscle or tendon pain temporarily.

When spread on the skin, analgesic ointments cause the blood vessels to widen, which increases the blood supply to the skin's surface. This reaction produces a warm feeling on the skin, but it does not hasten the healing process.

Q *Recently, I have heard many opinions about the safety of DMSO (Dimethylsulfoxide), a drug frequently used to treat muscle and tendon injuries in athletes. Why is this drug so controversial?*

A The Food and Drug Administration has not allowed the general use of DMSO because it neither hastens the healing process nor reduces swelling. DMSO weakens tendons, making them more susceptible to further injury. Furthermore, it has been reported to cause eye damage in laboratory animals.

DMSO does, however, reduce pain. In fact, it is such an effective pain reliever that the FDA condones its use in the treatment of the painful bladder condition, interstitial cystitis.

ICE-SKATING

Q *Is skating considered a fitness sport?*

A To strengthen your heart, you must exercise continuously. Skating is an ideal sport for fitness, because it requires that you continuously move one foot after the other. You glide on one foot while the other foot is in the air. As you start to lose momentum on that foot, you drop your other foot to the ice and glide on it.

Choosing the Proper Ice Skates

Q *Is there any particular formula for finding the correct size skates?*

A To get the maximum benefit and pleasure from ice-skating, you should choose your ice skates carefully.

Ice skates should fit snugly so the blades can function as an extension of your feet. If the boots are loose, you won't have full control of the blades. Then, when your ankle turns, you may find yourself skating on the side of your boot rather than on the blades.

To prevent this, you should select boots that are one size smaller than your street shoes. When shopping for skates, try on a pair, bang the back of the blade against the floor so that it will drive your heel snugly into the back of the boot, and lace up the skates all the way. Your big toe should reach the front of the boot.

Then stand. Make sure the boots feel snug, your ankles don't turn outward, and you can stand without wobbling. Although you want the boots to be snug enough to give you proper support, be sure they don't pinch your feet or your ankles. If they are too tight around your *malleoli* (the bumps on the outside and inside of your ankles) or around your feet, the boots may cause blisters or pain.

Also, choose boots that have a very stiff *counter,* the area that goes around the heel. To check them, press on the back of the boot, making sure there is little or no give.

When you're buying a pair of skates, make sure you wear socks that aren't too bulky since it is best to wear just one thin pair of socks when you skate. Wearing thick socks leaves so much space between your feet and the boots that you would have difficulty controlling the blades. Many players in the National Hockey League wear no socks under their boots. And, most female professional skaters wear pantyhose rather than socks.

JUMPING ROPE

Q *Is jumping rope an efficient way for me to improve my level of fitness? How does it compare to other workouts, say running?*

A Jumping rope is an excellent exercise for a number of reasons: it helps develop heart-lung fitness, it can be done indoors or out, and it is inexpensive. Depending on your speed, you can burn up to 600 calories an hour jumping rope. Nevertheless, although it looks easy, jumping rope is a demanding exercise that requires a high degree of physical fitness before you can exercise enough to strengthen your heart.

You must exercise at least 10 minutes continuously in order to strengthen your heart. But jumping rope for 10 minutes is difficult. To keep the rope from tangling, you have to spin it about 80 times a minute. And, jumping 80 times a minute is the equivalent of running a mile in seven minutes and 20 seconds. You have to be in very good shape to keep that pace for more than a few minutes.

If you are just beginning a regular exercise routine, begin gradually. It may take many months to get up to 10 continuous minutes of jumping rope. The best way to train is to use the *hard-easy principle*: one day, jump until your legs are heavy and then stop; the next day, jump for no more than two minutes. Continue this routine until you have reached your goal.

Q *Can you offer any special tips for someone like me? I'm in decent shape, but I'd like to begin jumping rope for nighttime and rainy-day exercise.*

A To begin your rope-jumping program, all you need is a rope. Sporting-goods stores sell special jump ropes with handles that let you spin the rope smoothly. Some even have digital counters to keep track of the number of times you jump. But, you can use any rope that fits your body. To assess this, stand on the middle of the rope and hold the ends up. They should just reach your armpits.

Q *What is the best type of shoes for a rope-jumping program?*

A You don't need expensive running shoes for indoor rope-jumping. In fact, you don't need any shoes at all. When you jump rope, you jump from your toes and land on your toes, so you don't need any padding on your heel. You should, however, bend your knees a bit when you land to absorb the shock as your toes hit the floor. And bend forward at the waist a little to help maintain your balance.

PUNCHING A BAG

Q *I was told by a friend who is an avid amateur boxer that hitting the jogging paths and doing laps in a pool aren't the only ways to reach and maintain fitness. He said I can achieve the same goal without risking injury by doing something as easy as hitting a punching bag three times a week. Is this true?*

A Lightweight air-filled bags are available at most sporting-goods stores. Unless you're an unusually hard puncher, you should be able to buy a bag for less than $200. Most of these bags are supported by a metal stand that is placed on the floor, or you can attach them to a sturdy wall. You may also want to buy leather punching gloves, since bare-handed punching can cause scrapes and blisters.

To begin your routine, hit the bag slowly enough with one hand so you can hit it again with your other hand when the bag bounces back toward you. If you keep your eyes on the bag and punch it so that you move continuously, you can get an excellent workout. In addition to reaching the necessary aerobic workout level—raising your heart rate to 120 beats a minute for 30 minutes—hitting a punching bag will help you burn calories. A person weighing 150 pounds burns 100 calories per half hour while punching a bag, the same amount of calories burned during a half-hour walk.

Stop as soon as your arms feel heavy or hurt, or you feel

tired. Don't start out doing 30 minutes of exercise. Instead, work up to it gradually.

This sport is a safe way to become fit because it places very little stress on the muscles and tendons in your arms. It also is extremely effective because exercising your arms instead of your legs makes your heart work harder for the same amount of effort. The blood vessels in your arms are smaller than those in your legs and offer greater resistance against the flow of blood. When you exercise vigorously using your arms, your heart must work 2½ times as hard as it does to pump the same amount of blood through your legs.

Q *Can women benefit from punching a bag?*

A Hitting a punching bag is good exercise for women as well as men, since it does not require a great deal of strength. Many people have found the sport helps improve their eye-hand coordination, which boosts their performance in other weight-loss sports such as racquetball and handball.

ROLLER-SKATING

Q *How much exercise can I get from roller-skating and how does it compare to other sports fitness-wise?*

A If you're looking for a fun way to get fit and lose some weight, try roller-skating. Skating is popular and convenient, in addition to being good exercise. Some 30 million Americans roller-skate regularly and they have more than 5,000 indoor rinks to choose from. Chances are that no matter where you live, you can find a place to skate year-round.

In just 30 minutes of skating you can burn 225 calories, about the same number burned during 30 minutes of aerobic dancing.

Almost 300,000 pairs of roller skates are purchased in this country every week! When many of us were kids, we wore metal skates that cost less than $10 and could be attached to our shoes. When steel wheels touched the pavement, our neighbors could hear us coming a block away.

Today, good roller skates have built-in boots and usually cost $100 or more. They have polyurethane wheels that can barely be heard as you skate by. Such skates are available with indoor or outdoor wheels. As a general rule, outdoor wheels are larger and softer; they must give with the roughness of the pavement. Indoor wheels usually are harder so they can grip the smooth wooden surface of an indoor rink.

The best boots are made from leather. They conform well to the shape of your heel and don't trap moisture.

When shopping for roller skates, make sure the boots fit your heels tightly.

A modern roller-skate boot has a toe-stop, a small wheel attached to the front plate just beneath the sole. If you want to stop suddenly, point your toe down. The friction between the toe-stop and the ground will act as a brake.

Be careful if you haven't skated since you were very young. Slowly build up your ability to skate for 10 continuous minutes and then work up to 30 minutes.

Take a few sensible safety precautions to prevent bumps, bruises, and broken bones. Wear a bicycle helmet and pads for your knees and elbows. This equipment is available at most sporting goods stores.

How to Roller-Skate

Q *Would you advise me to buy a big pair of boot skates if*

I am to take up roller-skating on a regular basis? Can I learn with a pair of old-fashioned metal skates?

A Boot skates give you much more control than the metal kind that attach to your shoes. To get the maximum control over your skates, make sure they're a size smaller than your shoes and wear them without socks.

The proper motion in roller-skating is from side to side. As you glide, your rear leg should be at a slight diagonal rather than straight back, and your front foot should be straightforward rather than turned out. This allows you to skate on the outside of your skates, which creates the right amount of friction to propel you forward in a smooth, gliding motion.

Your knees should be bent while you skate, but don't lift them as high as when you walk. If you lift them slightly, you'll achieve a continuous gliding motion and will have little trouble with your balance.

The more you lean forward, the faster you'll glide, so beginners should skate with their backs relatively straight.

As an added benefit, roller-skating is good preparation for other sports such as water-skiing, snow-skiing, and bicycling. When you roller-skate, your quadricep muscles in the front of your upper legs are worked as much as your hamstring muscles in the back of your legs. If you roller-skate enough, these sets of muscles will be almost equal in strength, a requirement for these other sports as well.

ROWING MACHINES

When spring weather is blustery and forbidding, many people look for a good indoor exercise to keep them fit. Pulling on a rowing machine can be that exercise. It is an excellent means of getting fit and staying that way.

Q *Where can I purchase a rowing machine to use at home?*

A At most sporting-goods stores. A good rowing machine consists of a metal bracket with a movable seat and two oars that move only forward and backward, not sideways. The machines cost from $200 to $500. With your own equipment, which is usually no larger than four feet by two feet, you can even row in your living room or bedroom while watching TV!

Make sure you buy a rowing machine with a movable seat. The increased circulation of blood caused by the entire rowing activity is what helps strengthen your heart and cardiovascular system. If the seat on the machine does not move, all you will be doing is moving your arms, and your heart will not be forced to pump enough blood to make it stronger.

When you row on a machine with a movable seat, you use your legs, arms, and back. For this reason, rowing is one of the best exercises for strengthening your back muscles.

Q *What is the correct technique for using a rowing machine?*

A Rowing your way to fitness is easy. Start by sitting in the machine, putting your feet in the stirrups, and bringing the seat all the way forward. Your knees will be bent and your upper body should be bent as far forward as possible. Grasp the oar handles in your hands and hold them close to your body. Start to row by straightening your knees, which pushes the seat backward. Then, start moving your upper body backward using your back muscles. Complete the maneuver by pulling the oars back. Work your feet, back, and arms—in that order.

RUNNING AND JOGGING

Almost 30 million Americans run, and nearly as many have questions about their sport. Some want to know how to avoid injuries, while others want to know how to deal with injuries they already have. Many runners seek ways to improve their speed or endurance, and others are merely trying to enjoy the sport. The running boom of the seventies and eighties has stimulated even more questioning than running, and these questions are reflected in the size of this section.

I hope the answers to many of your questions will be found in this section too.

Q *Is there really such a sport as "jogging" or are joggers simply slow runners?*

A Be careful whom you call a jogger, since most people who exercise in this way prefer to think of themselves as runners.

Jogging has a bad connotation. Jogging generally means running slowly. But, most people calling themselves runners claim to run a mile in between five and eight minutes. Few will admit to running slower than that. Despite these claims, however, it is usually only the serious, well-trained, competitive runner who moves faster than eight minutes a mile.

The National Jogging Association found out the hard way how many people react to the word jogging. Although the organization caters to recreational runners rather than hard-core competitive athletes, many members objected to being part of a group that had the word jogging in its title. They pressured the group into changing its name to the American Running and Fitness Association.

Q *What's the difference between a jogger and a runner?*

A I believe the true difference between a jogger and a runner lies in his or her motivation for hitting the road. Most joggers jog because they think it will give them longer, healthier lives. If they stop jogging, the only thing they miss is the sense of having gained potential health benefits. For runners, on the other hand, running is a significant part of their lives. If forced to stop running, these people often become depressed, irritable, and very difficult to live with. Scientists still aren't sure why this is so.

Jogging in Place

Q *Is jogging in place as effective as jogging on the roads to make you fit?*

A Yes. If you expend an equal amount of effort, you can burn the same number of calories, lose the same amount of body fat, and strengthen your heart as well by jogging in place as you would jogging outdoors.

You don't need any special equipment to jog in place. You don't even need to wear shoes, although it's advisable to jog on a rug to help cushion your landing.

In terms of fitness, jogging in place ranks high among exercises. The average jogger can burn 250 calories to 300 calories in 30 minutes. Jogging in place is also good for firming up muscles throughout your body.

But jogging in place will not strengthen your hamstring muscles (which are found in back of your upper legs) as much as jogging outdoors, since your hamstring muscles are used mainly to propel you forward. So, if you spend the winter jogging in place, you may have weak hamstring muscles and need to take it easy when you return to outdoor jogging.

For outdoor joggers, jogging in place is good exercise on your recovery days. For those of you who are out of shape, jogging in place is a good main exercise.

Running Shoes

Q *I know that running shoes can help to prevent injuries. I like to run in my bare feet. Is it safe?*

A If there are no rough stones or glass in your way, running on soft grass or sand can actually help protect you from injury. But, running barefoot on a hard surface such as asphalt, concrete, or wood increases your chances of injury.

When you run, you land on the outside part of the sole of your foot and roll to the inside. This motion helps cushion the force of your landing, distributing your weight so that your leg is better protected from injury than if you landed with full force on just one part of your foot.

But, the rolling-in motion also causes you to twist your lower leg inward, which can cause ankle, heel, knee, and hip injuries if there is nothing to control the movement.

Good running shoes should limit some of the rolling-in

motion, as will sand. When you run on sand, the exact imprint of your foot made by impact on the sand, provides support, thus limiting the inward motion.

Nevertheless, without support on a hard surface, your feet will tend to roll in excessively, significantly increasing your chances for injury. For running on a hard surface, always wear a running shoe that gives you maximum support.

Shoes for Narrow Feet

Q *I have very narrow feet, but the stores in my area carry running shoes only in a man's D width. Where can I get running shoes for narrow feet?*

A Go to a shoe store and have your feet measured. Then you can order running shoes in your exact width and length from Scarfo, 787 Boston Road, Bellerica, Massachusetts 01866; or New Balance, 38 Everett Street, Boston, Massachusetts 01866.

Training for Races

Q *I jog for 30 minutes every other day. Now I would like to start participating in races. How should I start?*

A To race, you have to run fast. However, each time that you run fast, your muscles are injured. You should allow at least one easy day to follow each fast day.

You will also need endurance. How long you can exercise a muscle is determined by how much sugar you can store in that muscle before you start to run. You increase muscle storage capacity by a process called *depletion*. Exercise until your muscles use up their stored muscle sugar. Then, when you eat a meal that is rich in carbohydrates (pasta, fruit, candy, cereal, beans), your muscles can hold more sugar than they could originally. Depletion is done not more than once a week.

Twice a week plan to run fast and once a week run long. The other four days are for recovery. Run slowly and for a short enough time so that you will be able to run fast or long on the next day.

Here is a typical training schedule for a beginner:

- Monday—Easy. Jog an easy two miles or try another sport.
- Tuesday—Hard. Run three miles very fast or do intervals (see next section).
- Wednesday—Easy. Jog two miles or try another sport.
- Thursday—Hard. Run seven miles hard or do intervals.
- Friday—Easy. Jog two miles or try another sport.
- Saturday—Easy. Rest.
- Sunday—Hard. Run 10 to 15 miles.

Intervals

Q *What are intervals and how do you do them?*

A In interval training, you run a fixed distance at a fixed pace for a set number of times with a fixed recovery period between runs. For example, instead of running a fast-paced three miles at one stretch, you can train by running one-quarter mile 12 times at 70 seconds each with an eighth of a mile jog for recovery between each interval.

Most people can't run quickly for long distances without injuring themselves; instead, they use interval training to help the brain to coordinate the body's more than 500 muscles at fast speeds.

You should limit the time period for your recoveries. Usually, this means jogging half the distance that you run in each fast interval. For example, if you are running quarter-mile intervals, jog one-eighth mile between each fast interval. If you feel tired after your recovery period, you are probably doing too many intervals or are running them too fast for your present level of conditioning.

Q *How do I put interval training to use for running a marathon?*

A If your aim is to run a marathon in three hours, or seven minutes per mile, you should run intervals at a faster pace than that. This means, for example, you'll run six intervals of one-half mile each at a pace of 2:45, or a 5:30 mile pace, which is 1½ minutes faster than your desired race pace. Your rest period should be a slow jog at half the distance. By training in short spurts, your body will adjust to running very fast. When you run the marathon, even if the distance slows you a bit from your training pace, you'll still reach your desired race pace.

To be effective, intervals should be run at least once but no more than three times a week. If you run intervals less than once a week, you won't prepare your body for speed. Doing them more than three times a week will leave you prone to injury.

Running Form

Q *I took up jogging six months ago and am thinking about racing. What kind of form should I use for racing?*

A In racing, you should take short strides, land on your heels, and keep your back straight.

The best runners take short strides. When you run, some of the force of your landing rebounds back to help propel you forward. If you take too long a stride you lose some of this rebound energy, or springing motion, and have to work much harder to maintain your speed.

Landing on your heels is preferable to landing on your toes because your leg muscles relax before pushing off from your toes for the next stride and are cushioned from the force of landing. If you land on your toes, your leg muscles are contracted for a longer period of time, which will tire you sooner.

Sprinters land on their toes because they're less concerned with fatigue than other runners. And, some of the best marathon runners, whose legs are stronger than their competitors', land on their toes when they race. In fact, in the last Boston Marathon, the top 10 runners all landed on their toes as they raced. But, most of the other runners landed on their heels.

Also, try to keep your back straight when you run on level ground or down hills. Leaning forward displaces your center of gravity so that you waste energy trying to keep yourself from falling.

On the other hand, when you run uphill you must lean forward to balance yourself because your center of gravity has already moved backward.

That Special Race

Q *I am a runner planning to enter a championship race this fall. How should I train so I can run my fastest time then?*

A In setting up a competitive athletic program, you need to start out with *background training*—running slowly to gradually increase your mileage. Then, about six weeks before your big race, decrease your mileage and run faster, a technique called *peaking*.

Be careful about your background training period. If you spend all your time running slowly, you will run slowly in your championship race, too. During this time, run most of your miles slowly, but also run faster once or twice a week.

As you get closer to your day of competition, try to run in some less important races at least once every week or two and increase the speed of your fast workouts. A few weeks before your championship race, you will be running so fast in some sessions that you won't be able to run too far.

Let your pre-championship races be your training guide. Say, for example, that you compete in the mile. In your first pre-championship race you run 4:50; in your second, 4:45; in your third, 4:38; and then, in your fourth, you run 4:55, a much slower time. This should tell you that you have passed your peak and need to slow down for a while. Go back to slow jogging for a week or two.

Running a Marathon

Q *I have run numerous 10K races in the past several years. Now I want to run the ultimate race, a marathon. Where do I start?*

A The first rule about running a marathon is to be sure you're ready for it. More and more people are entering marathons unprepared for the grueling distance, which is approximately 26¼ miles. That's why you'll see so many people at the end of many marathons come staggering across the finish line looking as if they need emergency care.

You should not run a marathon until you can run 15 miles on one day at a respectable pace—more than just a moderate jog—then recover enough to run hard and fast 48 hours later.

If you are ready to run a marathon, your preparation should include a carbohydrate-rich meal the night before the race. Loading up on such food as potatoes, bread, and pasta will improve your endurance.

Q *Is it advisable to drink water in longer races like the half-marathon or marathon?*

A In warm weather, you should make sure you drink cold water at frequent intervals. Don't wait until you feel thirsty, because by that time, you won't be able to replace the water you've already lost.

Q *Is there any special advice you give to people like me who are running their first marathon?*

A The most important advice I can give you is to start out more slowly than you think you should. In general, a fast start is the worst, and most common, mistake you can make.

When you get to the starting line, the prerace excitement will cause you to produce tremendous amounts of adrenalin, your body's own natural stimulant. This sudden rush of energy can make you think you can run faster than you really can.

Starting off too quickly will deplete your stored muscle sugar. Your muscles burn both fat and sugar for energy. When you run slowly, your muscles burn mostly fat. As you run faster, your muscles burn proportionately more sugar. When muscle sugar is depleted, your legs get heavy, your muscles ache, and you have problems with coordination. You won't feel the results of the loss of muscle sugar until you are more than 15 miles down the road—too late to refill your muscles with sugar.

You should use up your muscle sugar at a constant rate throughout the entire race. To do that, you should run an even pace.

Physical Characteristics for Speed

Q *What physical characteristics help a person run fast?*

A Oddly enough, flat-footed, pigeon-toed, bowlegged people are best equipped to run fast. Just stand by the starting line of a 100-yard dash. Most of the entrants will have those characteristics.

When you run, you land on the outside bottom part of your foot and roll to the inside. People with flat feet usually have normal arches, but their feet appear to be flat because they roll in excessively, causing their arches to touch the ground. Since flat-footed people usually roll in more than people with normal feet, they hit the ground with a greater force. That drives them forward with more force, so they run faster.

The strongest feet point inward in a pigeon-toed position. When you run with your toes pointed slightly inward, your feet are closer together and your heels do not slip backward, giving you a firmer landing and push-off. Running with your toes pointed outward, however, forces your heels to slip forward as you raise up on your toes before your feet leave the ground. This reduces the force of your push-off and slows you down.

Bow-legged people whip their knees inward as they step off from one foot to the other. This inward motion drives them forward, helping them to run faster.

So, a high school football coach can often pick his fastest halfbacks just by standing in the school corridor and looking for youngsters who are flat-footed, pigeon-toed, and bow-legged.

Jet Lag

Q *I plan to run a marathon in Australia next year. Will the change in time zones throw off my running?*

A Changing time zones certainly can interfere with athletic performance. Athletes flying long distances to the 1984 Olympics in Los Angeles had to contend with this when they crossed several time zones.

Everyone has a normal internal time cycle. We feel like getting up at a certain time and we eat and go to bed at certain times. Waking and sleeping cycles depend on body temperature. You fall asleep when your body temperature drops and you awaken when your temperature rises.

When your customary living times are disrupted, you may not feel well and may find it difficult to perform your usual tasks and to fall asleep. Some people develop constipation or diarrhea. For athletes, a change in time zones may affect their ability to compete at their best.

Several studies have shown that it takes at least 12 days for a person to adapt to a new time zone. So, my advice to you is to arrive in the city of your sporting event at least 12 days in advance. If you can't get to your destination that early, try the following technique while you're still at home: each night go to bed one or two hours later than you usually do until you reach the normal bedtime in the new zone. It doesn't work to try to go to sleep earlier—you'll just toss and turn.

Ankle Weights

Q *I plan to run a marathon in Australia next year. Will wearing ankle weights help me run faster?*

A Ankle weights can increase your chances of injury and will not help you to run faster or longer.

When you wear ankle weights, you must lift your legs with extra force to carry that weight. This lifting places more stress on the quadriceps muscle on the front of your upper leg. All muscles come in pairs, each one balanced by another that performs an opposite function. For example, the quadriceps muscles lift the knee while the hamstring muscles on the back of your upper leg lower the knee. Running with ankle weights can make the quadriceps too strong for the opposing hamstring muscle, increasing your chances of injuring the weaker of the pair.

Ankle weights won't help you run faster. Training is specific. To run fast in races, you must run fast during practice. Ankle weights slow you down during practice sessions, so they won't prepare you to run faster in races.

They won't help you run longer, either, because they will tire you earlier in your practice runs.

SKIING

You can use skiing for anything you want. If you want to become fit, try cross-country skiing. You'll have no trouble getting your pulse up beyond 100 beats per minute and you only have to ski for 10 minutes several times a week to begin strengthening your heart. If you like to move fast, just go down a hill. The only limit to how fast you go will be the depth and length of the hill—and, of course, your own courage!

Don't make the mistake of thinking you can easily become fit with downhill skiing. As you'll remember, you've got to work out continuously for at least 10 minutes for heart-lung fitness and to ski downhill continuously for 10 minutes takes a very long hill. Also, if you enjoy downhill skiing, don't make the mistake of doing it without adequate preparation. Downhill skiing is one of the most dangerous sports around and the forces on your muscles and tendons are tremendous. You shouldn't even try to ski until you strengthen the muscles, tendons, and ligaments that will be challenged most by skiing. We can't all ski on snow to prepare for skiing, but we can prepare by exercising the same muscles used in skiing through sports such as roller skiing or bicycling.

Buying Your First Pair of Skis

Q *I am ready to purchase a pair of skis after skiing several times with rental skis and discovering that I'd like to pursue the sport. How do I choose the correct pair?*

A Ideally, the length of your skis should equal the distance from the floor to the palm of your hand when you raise your arm straight above your head. Beginners find shorter skis easier to maneuver, however, because at slow speeds they are easier to control.

As important as length is the *camber* which is the slight curve in the middle of the ski. The camber ensures that your weight is distributed evenly along the length of the ski.

If the camber is too flexible, the middle part of your ski will dig into the snow and hinder your ability to execute turns. If the camber is too stiff, the front or rear of the ski will burrow into the snow, and you could fall.

The camber is rated soft, medium, and hard. Generally, those who weigh less than 125 pounds use soft. Skiers who weigh between 125 and 180 should consider a medium camber, and anyone over 180 should try a hard camber.

Preparing for Skiing

Q *I love to ski, but I live in Virginia and can only ski a few months a year. What's the best way to keep my body in shape for skiing?*

A If you can't ski often, the best way to keep yourself in shape for skiing is to use your muscles in the same way that you use them when you ski. This develops the same strength ratios for your muscles.

To do this, you could do something called roller skiing. Most sporting-goods stores sell special skis that have rollers attached to their bottoms; you use them by gliding along the roads using poles to propel you forward. You could also buy a special ski machine equipped with short skis that fit in tracks and a rope that you can pull on to imitate at home the motion of skiing.

For skiing, you need strong upper-leg muscles. You push the skis forward with your hips. Roller-skating and ice-skating and riding a bicycle also require strong upper-leg muscles. You glide when you roller skate or ice skate and, when you ride a bicycle, you push the pedals with your hip muscles. Jogging will not prepare you for skiing as well as roller or ice skating or pedaling a bicycle. Jogging stresses primarily your lower leg. When you jog, you land on your heel and then use the muscles of your lower leg to raise your body up on your toes.

World champion speed skater Eric Heiden provides a good example of the results gained from combining these sports. After winning five gold medals in Olympic speed skating, he was able to finish among America's top bicycle racers in competition after only 30 days of bicycle training. His muscles were prepared for cycling through skating. Sheila Young also was a world champion in both speed skating and bicycling.

Cross-Country Skiing

Q *I've heard that cross-country skiing is better for you than downhill skiing. Why is this so?*

A You strengthen your heart by exercising continuously for at least 10 minutes. Cross-country skiing is done continuously, while the time that you spend skiing downhill is limited by the length of the hill and the time that it takes to get back to the top.

Q *I am a runner who's recently switched to cross-country skiing. What mistakes in form might I have?*

A Unlike running, which requires a short stride, cross-country skiers need to take as long a stride as possible. Most of the force that advances you forward comes from pushing your front knee forward. The faster and farther you do so, the more efficiently you'll ski.

Another difference is posture. Runners run with their backs held straight, but skiers must lean forward. When you drive your poles into the snow the more you lean forward, the greater the force you can generate to propel yourself forward.

SWIMMING

What's the best sport for people who have arthritis, heart disease, obesity, or are just plain out of shape? Swimming would have to be one of the first answers that come to mind.

Swimming places a minimal stress on the joints due to the buoyancy of water. Swimming also places less strain on the heart, since it has to pump blood horizontally rather than vertically. If you are overweight, the water's natural buoyancy also tends to facilitate movement.

Swimming can be the easiest sport imaginable because you can tread water at such a slow rate. On the other hand, swimming can be as demanding as any other sport—if you push it. Just try swimming a few fast laps in a pool and you'll see how strenuous it can be.

Breathing During Swimming

Q *What is the proper way to breathe when I swim and how do I learn it?*

A Although most people enjoy swimming, many of them have problems breathing correctly. Sometimes they swallow water. At other times, they tire easily because they don't take in air properly. Once you learn the proper breathing technique in swimming, which is quite simple, you should solve both of these problems.

There are three principles to follow. First, hold your head in the water at hairline level. Second, breathe in shallowly, filling your upper chest instead of your entire chest cavity with air. Third, breathe in once each arm cycle.

Some people try to lift their head when they breathe, rather than turn it, which only wastes energy. If you keep your head in the water at hairline level, you'll encounter less resistance and increase your efficiency. To keep from swallowing water, just turn your head fully to one side so your mouth is above the waterline.

Breathing in shallowly conserves energy because you're using fewer muscles and exerting less force than when you breathe deeply. Aim for breathing naturally—not forcing in more air than you need. Your mouth will be above the waterline for only a few seconds so breathe in rapidly. Then, expel the air slowly; you have a longer time to breathe out when your face is in the water.

You need not breathe in more than once each arm cycle. If you breathe from the right side, you'll take a breath while your right arm is back and out of the water. Then you'll expel the air when your right arm is in the water.

Swimming Freestyle

Q *What does the term* freestyle *mean and how does it relate to the* crawl *stroke in swimming?*

A The crawl, or freestyle, is the most popular stroke in swimming, but many people are unable to swim the crawl continuously because they don't use their arms properly. In this stroke, your arms supply almost 100 percent of the force that drives you forward, while your kick's main function is to keep your body even in the water.

There is a science to swimming, and once you learn the basics of it, you'll move more efficiently through the water.

Each time your hand breaks the water, it should be placed in front of your head with your elbow bent. If you hold your elbow straight, your hand will enter the water too far out to the side, which will turn your body toward the opposite side rather than move you forward.

Your elbow should be higher than your hand at all times. The shoulder muscles that drive your arm down and back during stroking generate far more power in this position. Lowering your elbow below your hand limits the amount of force that can be transmitted from your shoulder muscles to your arms.

Contrary to what many people believe, you should not cup your hands. Rather, hold your fingers loosely together. Cupping decreases the surface area of your hand, which, in turn, limits the force of your hand as it moves through the water.

When your hand enters the water, put more effort into pushing your hand backward rather than downward. Pushing down raises your body up, and this bobbing motion will slow you down and tire you sooner.

Don't try to reach as far forward as you can when your arm enters the water. Instead, let your hand enter the water at a comfortable distance. When you reach far forward, you raise your shoulder blades, which limits the amount of power that your shoulder muscles can generate.

Use a firm, even stroke throughout. Varying the force provides an uneven acceleration and wastes energy. These techniques, which are used by competitive swimmers, can help anyone who wants to swim more comfortably for longer distances.

Q *I say that you kick to drive you forward. My coach tells me that the main function of a kick is to keep you going straight ahead. Who is right?*

A Your coach. The main function of a kick is to stabilize your body. It is supposed to keep your body from moving to one side or up or down.

When you stroke down with your left hand, the front part of your body moves to the right. You can limit this wasted motion by having your right foot enter the water at the same time as your left arm.

Stroking down with your arms also raises your upper body out of the water. To prevent this from happening, you should raise the leg on the same side of your body out of the water. For example, when you stroke down with your left arm, you should move your left leg up.

Q *Why do good swimmers keep their heads in the water when they swim the crawl?*

A To decrease the resistance of the water against your body. Since your head is narrower than your shoulders, it breaks the water with a smaller surface area and offers less resistance against the water. Airplanes have small noses for the same reason.

It is important to hold your head at the right depth. Since your head is round, less surface pushes against the water at your hairline.

Q *I notice that all top swimmers lift weights. Why do they do this?*

A Because you will swim faster if you increase your

strength. The harder that your hands press against the water, the greater the force with which they will drive you forward.

David Costill at Ball State University asked several swimmers to stop swimming and start working with special strength training machines that strengthened the arms by using the same motion employed in swimming. After several weeks of training for strength, the swimmers were timed in the water. They were able to go faster over short distances.

Q *I like to swim, but whenever I swim a lot I develop a painful infection in my ears. What causes this and how can I prevent it?*

A Swimmer's ear is usually due to an infection in the outer ear canal and is treated with antibiotic pills and ear drops. People who develop recurrent ear infections should insert dilute acetic acid drops into their ears each time that they come out of the water. These ear drops can be purchased at most drugstores.

Taking in Extra Oxygen

Q *I have often seen players on the sidelines at hockey or football games breathing from oxygen masks. Does inhaling oxygen help athletes catch their breath.*

A Swimmers who breathe hard and fast before a race or hockey players who take in oxygen from an oxygen tank before a game, are wasting their time. Taking in extra oxygen before you exercise or during breaks doesn't do any good and may actually harm you.

When you breathe, oxygen is carried into your lungs, crosses into your bloodstream, and then is carried to the rest of your body. When you're at rest, the blood vessels leading from your lungs are saturated with more than 98 percent of oxygen. You can do nothing to make them hold more oxygen—even if you breathe hard and fast to bring more oxygen into your lungs.

The only time the concentration of oxygen in the blood is lower than 98 percent is when an athlete is exercising full tilt. When he or she stops exercising, the concentration returns almost immediately to 98 percent.

You can see, then, that to benefit from breathing pure oxygen, a player would have to perform with a tank strapped to his or her back and a mask affixed to his or her face—all rather awkward. I assume that players take oxygen infusions on the sidelines because of some trainer's mistaken notion that this practice improves endurance and recovery.

The same principle applies when you stop exercising to take a break. It may be called "taking a breather," but while breathing from an oxygen tank will bring more oxygen into your lungs, it won't bring more of it into your bloodstream. And that means that your muscles won't get any more oxygen than they already have, so you won't be able to perform any better.

Q *When I'm out of breath after swimming for 20 to 25 minutes, will it help me to breathe extra hard for a minute or so?*

A Breathing in and out very quickly may actually harm you. You may hyperventilate because you're decreasing the amount of carbon dioxide in your body, which in turn increases your blood's alkalinity. When that happens, your muscles go into spasm.

Breathing pure oxygen can also have adverse effects because it causes your bronchial tubes to constrict. If you breathe pure oxygen and then start or continue to exercise, your contricted bronchial tubes prevent oxygen from getting into your lungs, which will cause your muscles to tire more easily.

However, during exercise, you can improve your performance by breathing deeply and taking in more oxygen. When you exercise, the oxygen levels in your bloodstream drop. Putting more oxygen into your lungs allows your blood vessels to absorb and then distribute more of it to the rest of your body, including your exercising muscles.

Hyperventilation

Q *My 11-year-old son is on his school's swim team. During a recent meet, as he stood on the starting block before a race, he had difficulty breathing and his muscles tightened up so he couldn't move. He was all right again within a few minutes, but I'm concerned. Can you tell me what happened?*

A He probably *hyperventilated*. This means he became nervous and started to breathe deeply and rapidly, which caused him to blow off excessive carbon dioxide from his lungs. His blood became less acid as a result. (Carbon dioxide is an acid-maker.) Muscles require a certain amount of acidity to be able to contract. When your son hyperventilated, all his muscles contracted at the same time.

Hyperventilation can be treated by putting a large paper bag over the victim's head for a moment so he will rebreathe some of his own carbon dioxide. Within seconds, his blood will return to its normal acidity and he can resume his activities.

Multiple Competitions in the Same Day

Q *As a swimming coach for youngsters who often com-pete in several events in one day, I don't know whether it is better to keep them moving after they finish an event or let them stop and rest. Which will best enable the swimmers to maintain their energy throughout the day?*

A If your swimmers are to compete in another race less than an hour after finishing one, it is better to keep them moving.

After participating in a hard race, a person's bloodstream is loaded with a breakdown product of exercise called *lactic acid*. Lactic acid accumulates in the bloodstream when there is a lack of oxygen. When the acid reaches high levels, it interferes with the normal chemical reactions of the muscles. This can make you tired and cause your muscles to hurt.

The faster lactic acid is cleared from the bloodstream, the quicker an athlete recovers. The most effective way to clear the bloodstream is to continue exercising at a slow, relaxed pace. Exercise speeds up the heart so that it pumps more blood. The blood then carries oxygen to the body's tissues. As soon as oxygen reaches the lactic acid, the acid breaks down.

Early to Bed

Q *I am a college sophomore who swims the backstroke on the swim team. Our coach always insists that we go to sleep early the night before a race, but I insist on my regular amount of sleep. Who is right?*

A Some coaches require their athletes to get to bed early on the night before a race. Many athletes believe in this ritual as a way to ensure their vitality the next day, whether for a game or a race. However, going to bed early will not necessarily mean you'll wake up refreshed. In fact, going to bed earlier than usual may leave you feeling exhausted the next morning.

How alert you are the next day depends on how deeply you sleep the night before, not on how many hours you stay in bed. If you're like most people, you've experienced times when you've spent many hours in bed tossing and turning and have woken up tired.

Going to sleep early defeats its own purpose because, unless you're tired, you won't sleep deeply. The last few hours that you're up are the ones that make you tired. By going to sleep early, you increase your chances of sleeping lightly throughout the night.

It's much wiser to stick to your regular sleep habits on the day before a competition. Your body will let you know when it's time to go to sleep.

Q *Will missing sleep harm me if I have an important race the next day?*

A Missing a night's sleep does not usually affect an athlete's performance. Even if you miss as many as three nights of sleep, you can still feel refreshed after you sleep about 12 hours to make up for the sleep you've lost.

If you go to bed later than usual and don't get much sleep on the night before a game or race, it probably won't affect your strength, speed, endurance, or coordination. You may feel tired, but once you get excited your body will produce enough adrenalin to stimulate you and make you alert.

Exercise helps promote deep sleep, so make sure you do some on the day before a competition. Exercise at a relaxed pace, not strenuously, and you should sleep deeply and be alert the day of the competition.

TENNIS

A lot of people think they can become fit by playing tennis. Unless they're very good tennis players, they are wrong. Remember that you need to exercise continuously for fitness, and most people can't volley continuously for any significant period of time. In fact, studies show that the average tennis player spends 80 percent of the time on court standing around waiting for the ball and burns less than 200 calories per hour. Compare that to brisk walking, which burns more than 300 calories per hour and you'll understand why tennis may not be the way to fitness.

Tennis is fun and requires a lot of skill, but if you're not a very good tennis player, you'll have to pick another sport for cardiovascular fitness. And, if you want to become strong, you'll have to lift weights or push on special strength machines.

Tennis elbow and *tennis leg* are muscle and tendon injuries that can be prevented by becoming strong *before* you go out on the court. To prevent tennis elbow, you should do special exercises to strengthen the muscles in your forearms; to prevent tennis leg, strengthen your calf muscles.

Preparing for Tennis

Many of you stop playing tennis in winter and then start playing it again in the spring. Remember that your body needs some conditioning before you begin playing.

Why? You've probably heard the horror stories of people who pull their calf muscles when they've come back to the tennis courts after not playing for a while. They leave themselves open for other injuries as well.

Q *How should I prepare myself for tennis so that I don't injure myself?*

A You can prepare your legs by jumping rope, running from side to side, and stretching the muscles in the back of your legs.

Spend a few minutes each day shifting your weight from side to side in a little run. Just jogging straight ahead won't develop your muscles in the same way that they are used when you play tennis.

And, since tennis players do a lot of jumping off their toes, jumping rope is excellent preparation for playing the game and is a good way to strengthen your leg muscles.

Q *Are there any stretches I can use especially for tennis?*

A Improving your flexibility may also help you prevent injuries. The most important muscles to stretch for tennis are the calf muscles in the back of your lower legs and the hamstrings in the back of your upper legs.

You can do this by performing wall push-ups and toe touches. For a wall push-up, stand three feet away from a wall with your arms outstretched and your palms against the wall at shoulder height. Bend your elbows while leaning your body closer to the wall, keeping your heels on the ground. Hold for 10 seconds. You should feel your leg muscles stretching. Keep bending and straightening your elbows slowly while keeping your feet firmly planted in the same spot.

To do toe touches, start by standing erect, then slowly bend your torso and try to have your fingers touch your toes. Hold for 10 seconds. Try not to bend your knees. If you can't touch your toes, don't force yourself. You can pull a muscle that way, and you won't be helping yourself. Slowly return to a standing position, then start the exercise again.

For a final conditioning, you ought to play a friendly game with the ball before you start slamming the ball by your opponent. Try hitting easy lobs until you feel ready to go out on the court.

Tennis Leg

Q *Not long ago, I was playing tennis when suddenly I heard a loud pop and felt like someone hit my lower leg with a stone. It was sore and stiff for a while, but seems better now. What happened, and what should I do if the injury occurs again?*

A It sounds as if you had a torn calf muscle, also known as *tennis leg*. Despite its name, this injury can occur when you are playing tennis or basketball, jogging, or doing any other exercise that involves running.

If your leg doesn't bother you anymore, it probably has healed without a doctor's treatment. Here's what you should do if it happens again.

First, as soon as you feel the pain, stop exercising. Sit down and elevate your injured leg. Then, apply something cold to the site where it hurts. Ice wrapped in a towel is best. Then, try to point your toes away from your body. If you can't do this, check with your doctor immediately. You may have a complete tear in the tendon and need surgery.

If you can point your toes, simply rest the leg for a few days. When you can stand on your toes without any pain, you can start to ride a bicycle to keep fit while your leg heals. Riding a bicycle stresses primarily the muscles in your upper leg. Again, if you feel any pain, stop exercising.

When you can walk without pain, resume your regular exercise regimen, but listen to your body and stop if your leg starts to hurt.

To prevent this injury from recurring, start calf-strengthening exercises. Here is a particularly good one: stand and slowly raise yourself on your toes. Then, slowly lower yourself. Do this 10 times, rest one minute, then do two more sets of 10. Do this every other day. When the toe raises are easy to do, try holding weights in your hands as you raise yourself on your toes. The added resistance will help to strengthen the calf muscles even more.

Tennis Elbow

Q *I'm suffering from tennis elbow. Will wearing a band over my elbow while I play tennis help me recover from the severe pain?*

A At best, wearing a band will keep your arm warm, but it won't help it to heal. To permit healing, you'll probably have to stop playing tennis for the time being and start exercising carefully.

Tennis elbow results from damage to the muscles and tendons that run from your wrist to your elbow. This damage occurs when the ball hits your racquet with greater force than your muscles can handle, causing your muscles and tendons to tear.

There are two types of tennis elbow: forehand and back-hand. To identify which one you have, stand with your arm to the side with your palm facing forward. If the pain is on the outside of your elbow, you've got backhand tennis elbow. If it's on the inside, you've got forehand tennis elbow.

You'll need to know which one you have before you start to exercise. With this knowledge you can identify the right way to perform exercises that will help to enlarge and strengthen those injured muscles and tendons.

For this exercise, which is one of the best for tennis elbow, you'll need a 2½-pound weight or dumbbell.

1. Sit next to a table, resting your lower arm on it.
2. Hold the 2½-pound weight in your fist.
3. Slowly raise your hand by bending your wrist and then lowering it. Here's where knowing which injury you have counts. If it's backhand tennis elbow, do this exercise with your palm down; if it's forehand tennis elbow, do it with your palm up.
4. Repeat 10 times.
5. Rest for one minute, then do two more sets of 10.

As you gain strength, increase the weight, never the number of repetitions.

TRAMPOLINES AND REBOUNDERS

Q *Is jumping on a trampoline considered a fitness exercise?*

A Remember the thrill you got as a child when you swooped through the air on a swing? You can get the same sort of "high" as an adult by jogging or jumping on a trampoline and get fit at the same time.

Trampolines have been around for a long time. The large trampolines got a bad reputation because many people were badly injured when they tried to do stunts. Recently, manufacturers have produced mini-trampolines, called *rebounders*, that are about three feet in diameter and are raised about one foot off the ground. They are sold in most sporting-goods and large department stores for $80 to $200. They are safer than the larger trampolines because they are too small for stunts.

First, some precautions. Jumping on a trampoline is harder on your body than walking or jogging; since you land from a higher position, you hit the mat with a much greater force. Jumping can aggravate back and other joint problems. Also, people over 40 should be careful when they jump, because aging causes their bones to lose calcium, making them more likely to break.

On the other hand, jogging on a trampoline is as good an exercise as jogging on the roads and is safer. Your foot strikes the mat with less than one-sixth of the force with which it strikes the ground. The mat gives with each step and absorbs some of the shock, so less force is transmitted to your body.

Q *I saw a device called a rebounder at the sporting goods store recently. It resembles a small trampoline. How can I use it to exercise?*

A To use a rebounder, stand in the middle of the mat with your bare feet. Start off by jogging or walking on the trampoline until your legs feel heavy or hurt or you feel tired. Then stop. Every other day, continue your routine, gradually working up to 30 minutes.

WALKING AND HIKING

If you're overweight and are looking for a sport to get you into shape, try walking. Approximately 44 million Americans say that their major exercise is walking. A regular regimen of walking strengthens your heart, burns a lot of calories, and is safer than almost any other exercise.

You will strengthen your heart by following the rules of strength training, namely, raising your heartbeat to 120 beats per minute each time you exercise, which should be at least 20 minutes a day, three days a week. Since walking is a relatively easy sport, you should have no problem meeting these goals.

Q *How does walking compare to running in terms of exercise?*

A Compared to running, walking is safer, and also burns calories more effectively in relation to mileage. When you walk, you must keep one foot on the ground at all times, which means that as you stride you hit the ground with a force equal to your body weight. The soft landing makes muscle injury unlikely. When you run, however, you momentarily have both feet off the ground at the same time, which means when you land, you hit the ground with a force of more than three times your body weight. The hard landing is a major cause of muscle injuries in runners.

When you run, you burn 100 calories per mile whether you run quickly or slowly. The faster you walk, however, the more calories per mile you burn. For example, you'll burn 56 calories per mile when you walk at the rate of 3 MPH, which equals about 20 minutes per mile (an average walking pace);

at 5 MPH, which equals about 15 minutes per mile (a fast pace), you'll burn 128 calories per mile.

Why the difference? No matter how fast you run, you use the same form; your hips face forward and your arms move very little. But, if you walk faster, your hips will swivel and your arms will swing more, which makes you burn more calories.

Q *What kind of shoes are best for walking?*

A The best shoes for walking are a good pair of running shoes. Their flexible soles will help you avoid heel pain, and they provide enough support to limit the rolling-in motion of your lower leg, which can cause hip, knee, and ankle pain.

As for form, the only thing you should strive for is gradually to take longer strides, which propel you forward faster.

On your first day out, try to walk at a brisk but comfortable rate. Walking slowly will not increase your heart rate enough to help you become fit.

Q *Ten months ago I started a walking program. I have built myself up so I can walk vigorously for 20 minutes with a heart rate of 120 beats a minute. Recently, I bought a stationary bicycle, but I can't ride for more than 5 minutes at the same heart rate I achieve when I walk. Why is this so?*

A Training for strength and endurance is specific. Walking strengthens primarily the muscles in your lower leg. Pedaling stresses the muscles in your upper legs. So, when you switched from walking to cycling, your upper leg muscles were not strong enough to continue pedaling for any length of time.

Don't be discouraged, though. The heart training effect from walking will carry over to your bicycle riding. If you persist in your exercise, you will quickly be able to achieve the same heart rate for the same length of time while bicycling.

Q *I have run for years without injury. Now that I am in my fifties, it seems that I am injured at least once a month. My wife says that walking is much safer than running and she wants me to walk with her. Why is walking safer than running?*

A It places far less stress on your body. During walking, you always have at least one foot on the ground, so the force of your foot striking the ground is equal to around one body weight. Just before your foot hits the ground during running, you have both feet off the ground so your foot strikes the ground with a force equal to around three times your body weight. This force is transmitted to your legs, knees, hips, and back, which increases your chances of injuring them.

Q *What's the most efficient way to walk?*

A Keep your back straight and your head high. Leaning

forward or backward displaces your center of gravity so you waste energy trying to keep yourself from falling.

Take long, comfortable strides. The longer strides cover more distance, so you move faster. This is different from running in which longer strides waste energy. When you run, more than two-thirds of the force of your footstrike is returned to drive you forward. When your heel strikes the ground, your muscles contract and pull the tendons tight, like rubber bands. This is stored energy. Then, when your foot comes off the ground, the tendons recoil to drive you forward. When you take very long strides during running, you lose some of the recoil force of your tendons and must use more energy to drive yourself forward.

Land on your heels when walking. Landing on your toes forces you to lean too far forward so you waste energy keeping yourself from falling.

Choosing Hiking Boots

Q *How can I choose hiking boots so that they fit properly?*

A Make sure that you get hiking boots at least a half or even a full size larger than your regular shoes. When you walk long distances, your feet swell and you should have enough room to accommodate the increased size. Another reason for the longer shoes is to accommodate thicker socks that absorb perspiration. When you hike, you will perspire profusely; walking in wet socks can soften and wear away the skin on your feet.

When you are at the shoe store, try the boots on and move your foot as far forward as possible. You should be able to get your thumb between your heel and the back of the boot. Next, lace them up and judge how they feel. If they don't feel comfortable in the store, don't buy them. They'll probably hurt you when you're on the trail.

Q *I like to go on long hikes on the trails with my family. After several hours of hiking, however, I frequently end up with raw, blistered feet. How can I prevent this?*

A Keep your feet dry. Wetness causes the skin on your feet to stick to your socks so the skin can be rubbed off or form blisters.

Always wear hiking boots that are larger than your street shoes. This allows extra space for thick socks and the swelling that naturally follows long hours of walking.

Wear thick socks with powder in the toes to absorb sweat. If you walk across a stream, make sure that you keep your socks dry. Take off your socks and boots, and then put your boots back on so the stones on the bottom of the stream don't cut your feet. Then, after you have crossed the stream, remove the boots, dry your feet and boots, and then put on your dry socks and boots.

If your feet start to hurt from tight shoes, chances are that your feet have swollen with fluid. Stop hiking, take off your boots, and lie with your feet above your heart. Gravity will take the extra fluid out of your feet so that your boots will fit when you replace them.

If you develop a blister, stop walking and take off your shoes and socks. Then, clean off the area around the blister with alcohol or any other antiseptic that you may have. Use a sterile pin to puncture the skin overlying the blister at its side. Then, use your thumb to express the fluid, being careful not to tear the skin overlying the blister. Cover the blister with white tape to make the skin overlying the blister adhere to its base.

5

SOME QUESTIONS AND ANSWERS ABOUT STRENGTH TRAINING

HOW YOU DO IT

You can't train for great strength and for heart and lung fitness at the same time. You've already learned that you strengthen your heart by exercising continuously for *at least 10 minutes.* You strengthen your skeletal muscles by exercising for *not more than 50 consecutive seconds.*

The only way to make a muscle stronger is to exercise it against resistance. Physiologists call it *stretching during contraction.* For example, when you try to lift a very heavy weight, your muscles contract before the weight starts to move. This causes the fibers to stretch. The more they can stretch without tearing, the greater the gain in strength.

To become strong, you want to strengthen as many muscle fibers as possible. The first time that you lift a heavy weight, you use only a few fibers; the second time, you use a few more. With each successive lift, you use more fibers until large amounts of lactic acid start to build up in your muscles. Then you use fewer fibers. It takes from about 30 to 50 seconds for significant amounts of lactic acid to build up in your bloodstream. In that time, you can lift and lower a heavy weight slowly 8 to 12 times.

To become strong, you should pick 10 to 15 different exercises that concentrate on different muscle groups throughout your body. Choose the heaviest weight that you can lift comfortably and use it 10 times in each exercise. Do this every other day, increasing the weight as you can.

ADVANTAGES OF BEING STRONG

Q *Lately, health-club advertisements have been extolling the virtues of strength-training machines to help us develop large, strong muscles. But, are there any advantages in having big muscles?*

A The larger your muscles, the more calories it takes for you to do your daily tasks. For example, if you weigh 150 pounds, you will burn 60 calories by walking one mile. But, if you put on an extra 20 pounds of muscle, you will burn 10 more calories per mile, or 70 calories. Over the course of a day, the extra muscle will help you burn hundreds of extra calories without doing much extra exercise.

The extra strength you gain when you enlarge your muscles helps you perform routine tasks such as using a hammer, sawing, turning a screwdriver, changing an automobile tire, opening a stuck door, or just opening a bottle.

NEGATIVE LIFTING

Q *I've heard weight lifters talk about negative lifting. What is it, and does it make you stronger?*

A In *negative lifting*, also known as eccentric contractions, instead of raising and lowering a weight you only lower it. You start with your arms raised, someone places weights in your hands, and you lower them. Negative lifting can make you stronger, but it also is more likely to injure you.

You can lower much heavier weights than you can lift. Some weight lifters can lower as much as 40 percent more weight than they can lift. For example, a weight lifter who can bench press 200 pounds can probably lower about 280 pounds.

The more you stretch a muscle without tearing it, the more you gain in strength after the muscle heals over the following 48 hours. Since the heavier weights offer greater resistance, you can gain more strength by negative lifting than by regular weight lifting. But, the greater resistance also increases your risk of tearing your muscle fibers. So don't do negative lifting more often than once a week.

STRENGTH FOR FOOTBALL

Q *I am a tackle on my high school football team. What is the best way for me to become stronger?*

A I'd suggest doing squats—deep knee bends—with very heavy weights on your back. This exercise reproduces the same explosive force you need to push opposing linemen out of your way.

Each muscle is composed of many small fibers. You want not only to strengthen each individual fiber, but to learn to contract simultaneously as many of the muscle fibers as possible, thereby increasing the total force of the muscle itself.

Perhaps you have heard of the story of a 98-pound woman who, in an emergency, lifted a 2,000-pound car that had rolled over on her husband? Although she may not have been particularly strong, she was able to contract most of her individual muscle fibers at the same time, which gave her enormous strength.

The use of the weights helps strengthen the individual muscle fibers. And, repeating the explosive motion of the squat educates your muscle fibers to work in the same way that you would use them to push aside an opposing lineman.

STRENGTH TO HELP YOU JUMP HIGHER

Q *Is there any type of weight lifting that will help me to improve my jumping ability?*

A If you participate in a sport in which you need to jump— basketball, high jumping, or figure skating, for example— special exercises will help you jump higher.

Each muscle is made up of thousands of small, stringy fibers. There are two ways to become stronger: one is to increase the size of the muscle fibers; the other is to learn to contract a greater number of fibers at the same time. The latter is most important in training your body to jump higher.

You can use weights or any strength-training exercise to make the fibers become larger. But, to teach your brain to contract a greater number of fibers simultaneously, you must do strength-training exercises that work your muscles in the same way that they are used when you jump.

Most people are able to contract about 10 percent to 30 percent of their muscle fibers at the same time; champion weight lifters can contract about 50 percent to 70 percent. Your aim is to contract as many fibers together as you can, since the more you contract, the more force you will exert against gravity and the higher you will jump.

Exercising with freestanding heavy weights on your shoulders can help you jump higher. So can using jump-training machines that place a heavy resistance on your shoulders while you raise yourself from a squatting position. These machines are found in most gyms and health clubs. In either case, use the heaviest weight you can lift eight times. When trying to ascertain which weight that is, don't start off with a heavy weight. Instead, test yourself by starting with a light weight. Then, gradually increase the weights until you find the right one.

First, stand with the weights on your shoulders. If you are using freestanding weights, you'll have to hold them firmly in place with your hands. Lower your body by bending your knees, then straighten them to stand erect. Do this eight times. You should do this every other day, and not more than three times a week.

As you get stronger, you will be able to do the exercise more than eight times. When you can lift the weights 12 times, increase the weights by about 10 pounds. Repeat the cycle, increasing the weights in 10-pound increments.

STRENGTH-TRAINING EQUIPMENT

Q *I'd like to become stronger but I can't afford to join an expensive club with weight-training equipment. What's the* *least expensive way I can get into strength training?*

A For less than $300, you can buy an inexpensive 110-pound barbell set (less than $50), a squat rack (about $100), and a bench (about $100).

You can strengthen many of your muscles by using just the barbell set and no other equipment. But, a complete strength program also should include squats for your legs, bench presses for your upper body, and tricep extensions for your arms.

When you do a squat, place the heavy barbell across your shoulders, squat down, then raise yourself. The weights will feel so heavy that after you finish you may not be able to move the weights from your shoulders. A squat rack will solve that problem. It includes a pair of posts set so they can hold the barbell at the same height as your shoulders. After you finish your squats, back up to the posts and place the barbell on the rack.

To strengthen your upper body without stressing your back, lie on a weight bench and press the weighted barbell up from your chest. Weight benches also have special posts to hold the barbell after you finish lifting it.

ISOMETRICS

Q *Are isometric exercises a good way to become strong?*

A To make a muscle stronger you must exercise it against resistance. Since in isometrics you push against an immovable force, such as a wall, you can certainly become very strong by doing isometric exercises.

Isometric exercises, however, have two drawbacks. First,

they can cause your blood pressure to rise to very high levels and, second, they make you stronger only in a limited way.

Your blood pressure rises when you exercise against resistance, especially during isometrics. When you push against an immovable object, your muscles contract and squeeze the blood vessels so that your blood pressure must increase tremendously to circulate blood through the squeezed arteries. Blood pressures as high as 300/250 have been recorded during isometric contractions. This squeezing of the muscles is more sustained in isometric exercises than in other resistance exercise. Therefore, it's best to avoid isometric exercise if you have high blood pressure or heart trouble.

The strength gained during isometric contractions is limited to the angle at which you hold your joints. Thus, if you push against a wall with bent elbows, your muscles will become stronger while your elbows are bent, but not when your arms are straight. Exercises that involve moving against resistance, such as weight lifting and pushing on a strength-training machine, can make you stronger both while you bend and straighten the joints.

TRAIN FOR STRENGTH AND FITNESS

Q *What is the best way to train for fitness and strength at the same time?*

A If you want both strength and cardiopulmonary fitness, you'll need to alternate strength-training exercises with continuous exercise. You can do both on the same day. For example, run in the morning and lift weights or work on strength-training machines in the afternoon and rest the following day. Or, you can alternate your activities—run one day and lift weights the next.

Never do strength-training exercises on successive days. When you lift weights or push on strength-training machines, your muscle fibers are slightly damaged. When they heal, they are stronger than before, but healing takes about 48 hours.

Also, most of us develop muscle soreness 8 to 24 hours after we exercise. You'll ache if you do the same sport with the same intensity during that time. If you alternate your choice of activity, however, and use your muscles differently, you probably can recover while you continue exercising.

Some people claim they can do strength training on the lower body one day and on the upper body the next. But, it is impossible to exercise an isolated part of your body during strength training; it stresses your entire body, whether you feel it or not.

MUSCLE-BOUND

Q *I'm a 26-year-old female runner interested in weight training to strengthen my upper body. Will this exercise make me muscle-bound, slow, and less flexible?*

A Lifting weights and pushing on the special strength-training machines found in many health and fitness clubs and gyms will make you stronger, faster, and more flexible.

To be "muscle-bound" is supposed to mean that you lose your coordination as a result of overly enlarged muscles. But, there is no such thing as being muscle-bound. Dexterity is a function of your brain's ability to coordinate your muscles and, no matter how large your muscles get, they will not interfere with that function.

Each of your muscles is composed of thousands of tiny fibers that fall into two types: fast-twitch, which govern strength and speed, and slow-twitch, which govern endurance.

When you work out to become stronger, you train the same muscle fibers that help you become faster.

Strength training won't make you any less flexible. To become flexible, you must stretch your muscles. When you lift heavy weights or push on strength-training machines, your muscles stretch before the weights begin to move. So, strength training will make you more flexible, not less.

DO MUSCLES TURN TO FAT?

Q *Is it true that if a person who exercises a lot and gets large muscles later stops exercising, the muscles will turn to fat?*

A This is an extremely common misconception, but it is nonsense. Muscles cannot possibly turn to fat.

When you exercise, your muscles often become larger and stronger. Muscles contain protein, which is composed of *amino acids*, or building blocks. The amino acids constantly travel out of the muscles into the bloodstream and then back into the muscles. This happens whether or not you exercise. Exercise, however, is a major stimulus to drive the amino acids into the muscle tissue at an increased rate. As a result, the muscles become larger and stronger.

If you are a regular exerciser and you suddenly stop exercising, there is less stimulus for the amino acids to return to the muscles, which become smaller.

Instead, the amino acids go into your bloodstream and, since your body has no way to store extra protein after it is released by your muscles, the amino acids are broken down into ammonia and organic acids that are then eliminated in your urine.

The only way you will become fat after you stop exercising

is if you continue to eat as much as you did when you exercised and were burning more calories. But, that has nothing to do with the size of your muscles. That has to do with eating too much. Solution: don't stop exercising.

TIRED MUSCLES

Picture this: the coach of a National Football League team vying for a bowl title is pacing the sidelines while the network TV cameras are trained on him. He is talking strategy with his coaching staff as a long third quarter plays out on the stadium clock.

His best kicker has a sore leg from an injury suffered earlier in the season and has already kicked five or six times today. A younger, less-experienced kicker sits waiting on the bench.

The dilemma: should the coach use the fresh, but inexperienced kicker in the closing quarter of the game, or should he rely on the exhausted, but better kicker?

In this situation the fresh kicker may do better.

Since 1939, we've known that how long you're able to exercise a muscle depends on how long you can keep stored sugar in it. In other words, endurance depends on your muscle sugar supply. But only recently has it been shown that, you also lose strength and speed when your muscles are low in their stored sugar supply.

When you exercise vigorously and use up part of your stored muscle sugar, or *glycogen*, you will not be able to generate as much force to kick hard, jump high, or throw far as you would when your muscle were fresh and filled with glycogen.

When a muscle's glycogen supply is depleted, the muscle becomes uncoordinated and aches. Glycogen cannot be transferred from one muscle to another, so it is not possible for your tired muscles to draw new glycogen from other, less stressed muscles. That's why the muscles you exercise the hardest run out of glycogen first and tire quickest. For example, a quarterback's throwing arm may give out before his legs.

All muscle fibers depend primarily on their stored sugar supply for energy. Your muscles contain two major types of fibers: a fast-twitch fiber to control strength and speed and a slow-twitch fiber to control endurance. During hard, exhaustive exercise—such as a long football game—fast-twitch fibers run out of stored glycogen long before the slow-twitch ones do. Because fast-twitch fibers are used to kick a ball, the exhausted kicker who has played hard throughout the football game has depleted much of the sugar stored in his fast-twitch fibers and will not be able to kick as far as he did earlier. This principle applies to all athletic maneuvers that require strength and speed, including kicking in soccer, jumping in basketball, and hitting slap shots in hockey.

TREATING MUSCLE INJURIES

Q *What is the best way to treat a muscle injury?*

A Muscle injuries, including those that occur during athletic competition or training, are best treated by rest followed by strengthening.

When you first injure a muscle, you should rest it so the torn fibers can heal. If you tear the calf muscle in the back of your lower leg, for example, stop any sports activity (such as running) that stresses the calf. Switch to another activity that will not stress the injured part. Riding a bicycle is a good alternate sport while you are recovering from a calf injury because cycling puts little stress on the lower leg.

After a few days, stand and try to raise yourself from your

heels to your toes. When you can do this without pain, you are ready to start strengthening the calf muscle. Stand and slowly rise to your toes, then slowly lower yourself. Stop if you feel any pain. Repeat the process 10 times (one set). Rest for a minute and do two more sets. Perform this exercise every other day. When you can do three sets with ease, try doing them while holding a weight (such as a barbell) in your hands. As you become stronger, increase the amount of weight.

The same rules apply to other muscle injuries such as a pulled hamstring—a muscle in the back of your upper leg. Stop any exercise that strains the hamstring and switch to an alternate sport such as swimming. When you are ready to strengthen the hamstring, attach a weight to the foot of the injured leg. To do this, use a weighted boot, which can be bought at most sporting-goods stores for about $20. These special boots have an area for attaching weights as well as straps to keep them in place. Stand straight and slowly bend the knee of the injured leg, raising the heel back so it moves toward your buttocks. Slowly lower your foot. Then, slowly straighten the knee. Do this 10 times (one set). Rest a minute and do two more sets. Do three sets every other day. As you become stronger, increase the weight on your foot.

DEEP KNEE-BENDS

Q *Are deep knee-bends dangerous?*

A Deep knee-bends place a lot of pressure on your legs and lower back and can cause injury if you don't use proper equipment and techniques. They are done by raising yourself from a squat position while working against heavy resistance placed on your neck and shoulders. A barbell or special weight-training machine can provide the resistance.

Before you start, strap a thick leather belt around your waist to support your lower back and place special triangular blocks under your heels to help keep you from leaning forward.

The safest way to do deep knee-bends is to use a machine that holds the weight above the floor. It will relieve the pressure from your shoulders as you lower yourself after each lift. You could also use a special barbell rack or have two strong friends nearby to hold the ends of the barbell when you have finished your squats.

Inexperienced lifters can protect their knee joints by placing a chair under their pelvises. If they slip, they will sit on the chair instead of falling to the floor with the weight on top of them.

Always keep your back straight during deep knee-bends. Squat and raise yourself by slowly straightening your knees. If you feel you are losing control, immediately raise yourself to a standing position before you slip or fall.

HOW TO DO SIT-UPS CORRECTLY

Q *I have seen people do sit-ups in any number of ways. What is the correct method for maximum benefit and minimum risk?*

A Sit-ups are excellent for strengthening and firming stomach muscles. But if they are not done correctly they could increase your chances of developing back pain.

Sit-ups should be done while you lie on your back with your knees bent enough for the soles of your feet to rest on the floor. Place your hands behind your neck. Slowly raise your head off the ground. Next, slowly raise your shoulders about 10 inches off the ground. You needn't raise yourself higher. Gradually lower yourself back to your original position.

Repeat this exercise 10 times. Rest a minute, then do two more sets of 10 sit-ups.

When you've been doing the sit-ups long enough for them to feel easy, wrap a towel around an object that weighs from two to five pounds and hold this weight in your hands behind your neck as you do the exercise. As your stomach muscles become stronger, you can increase the weight.

Keep your knees bent during sit-ups. Keeping your legs straight forces you to lift your weight with the *iliopsoas* muscle, which runs from the top of your leg bone to the inside of your pelvis. Straight-leg sit-ups strengthen and shorten the iliopsoas and increase the curve in your lower back, which, in turn, increases your chance of developing back pain.

Sit up only about 10 inches, because raising yourself higher forces you to use your quadriceps muscles in the front of your upper legs instead of your abdominal muscles. Strengthening and shortening these muscles also increases your chances of hurting your lower back.

Because bent-knee sit-ups can aggravate some disk problems, be sure to check with your doctor before doing this exercise.

THE HAMSTRING MUSCLE

Q *I play halfback on my college football team. Three times in the past three years I pulled my hamstring muscle. Why does this happen to me repeatedly?*

A Hamstring muscles, which are located in the back of your upper legs, usually are torn because the force exerted on them during exercise is greater than their inherent strength. People who participate in sports that require running have stronger *quadricep* muscles (located in the front of the upper leg) than hamstring muscles. Most people who develop pulled or torn hamstrings have quadricep muscles that are more than 1½ times as strong as their hamstring muscles.

When you first feel pain in your hamstring muscles, you should immediately stop playing football. Further exercise will only tear more muscle fibers, causing you more pain. In a few days, you should be able to walk without feeling pain. That's when you should start strengthening your muscles to protect yourself from pulling your hamstrings again.

You need to strengthen the weaker hamstring muscles and stretch the quadricep muscles. To stretch your quadricep muscles, stand on one leg and, bending the knee of the opposite leg, hold that ankle against your buttock for the count of 10; then relax. Repeat five times on each leg.

To strengthen your hamstring muscles, attach a weight to one foot. Standing on the other foot, slowly raise the weighted foot in back of you by bending your knee, then lower it by straightening your knee. Repeat 10 times, rest one minute, and do two more sets of 10; then repeat the entire procedure with the other leg.

6
SOME QUESTIONS AND ANSWERS ABOUT FLEXIBILITY TRAINING

Q *Can you explain how I can improve my flexibility?*

A Flexibility is very important for athletes because it improves athletic performance and helps prevent injuries. For most sports, you can increase your flexibility enough by doing specific stretching exercises. But, athletes who require a great deal of flexibility, such as gymnasts and divers, and people who have suffered injuries because they lack flexibility and who must rehabilitate their muscles, may need another, more effective means of achieving maximum flexibility.

In that method, you heat a muscle while stretching it, hold the stretch for 10 to 15 minutes, and then cool the muscle before you release it from the stretch. This is especially effective for stretching your Achilles tendons or your hamstring muscles.

Muscle temperature is important because it is easier to

stretch a warm muscle than a cold one. Rapid cooling of the muscle before relaxing it helps retain the stretch.

Q *What's the most effective way to heat or cool down a muscle?*

A When someone goes through rehabilitation, physicians and physical therapists use several different means of heating a muscle, including ultrasound waves and infrared lamps.

To use this method on your own, you may stretch while you're in a warm bath, or you may apply a warm-water bottle or a hot pack (a chemical package found in most pharmacies) on the muscle being stretched. Water heated to 108°F will raise your muscle temperature to around 105°F after at least 10 minutes.

Once you've stretched the muscle for the required amount of time, rapidly cool it before you release it from the stretch by applying an ice pack to the muscle for a few moments. Then relax the muscle. You'll be as stretched as possible.

But, even this maximum stretch doesn't last more than a day, so if you need maximum flexibility, you should use this method daily.

POSTURE AND BACK PAIN

Q *What is the relationship between poor posture and lower back pain?*

A When you were a child, your teacher may have graded

your posture and checked the curve in your back by placing one hand on your stomach and the other hand on your back. If your lower back was deeply curved, you failed the test. If your back and stomach were flat, you received a good grade.

Your teacher probably was most concerned about your posture for the sake of appearances. But, good posture can also mean better health. Many people with poor posture have deeply curved lower backs and suffer from lower back pain. People with good posture often avoid that problem.

Incidentally, your teacher may have believed that good posture required you to hold your head up straight and your shoulders back. There is no evidence that this position prevents back pain or improves your health. What does matter is the tilt of your pelvis. If it tilts forward too much, sticking your buttocks out, the curve in your lower back is exaggerated. This exaggerated curve may cause strain of the muscles and ligaments that hold together your spinal column. This can be very painful to your lower back.

If you have a deep curve in your lower back and feel pain there, your doctor may recommend exercises to correct the forward tilt of your pelvis. To do this, you must stretch your lower back muscles and strengthen your stomach muscles. Here are three good exercises:

Mild lower-back stretch (increases lower back flexibility): lie on your back with a small pillow under your head. Bend your knees at a 45-degree angle with your feet flat on the floor. Next, put both hands on your lower right leg, just below the knee, and pull the knee toward your chest. Hold for 10 seconds. Then slowly lower your leg. Repeat with left leg. Do this exercise 25 times with each leg.

Leg raise (strengthens stomach muscles): lie on the floor with your hands palms-down under your buttocks to help support your lower back. Bend your knees slightly with your heels on the floor. Keeping your knees bent and the small of your back touching the floor, slowly raise both legs until your thighs are at a 90-degree angle to the floor. Then slowly lower your legs. Do 8 leg raises and work up to 20. *Note:* Doing this exercise with your legs straight may strain your lower back.

Pelvic tilt (strengthens your stomach muscles and stretches lower back muscles): lie on your back with your knees bent and your feet flat on the floor. Press the small of your back into the floor and tighten your buttocks. Put your weight on your heels, keeping the small of your back flat. Then, raise your hips one inch off the floor and hold for 10 seconds. Then lower your hips and relax. Repeat 10 times.

TOE TOUCHING

Q *Is toe touching dangerous?*

A Touching your toes while standing straight is a good exercise to strengthen your leg muscles and make them flexible. If you have a rigid back, however, this exercise could injure you.

When you reach for your toes, you bend at the hips. When you have bent as far as you can at the hips and try to go farther down, you must arch your back. If your back is flexible and you bend easily at the hips, you'll have no trouble touching your toes.

If your hips restrict your bending motion or if your back is rigid, you could tear the muscles and ligaments supporting your back. It's far safer for you to touch your toes while sitting down.

Here are two ways to do that:

Leg stretch #1: sit upright on the floor with your legs spread apart in front of you. Point your toes. Slowly stretch both arms forward toward your left foot. Bend your head down toward your left knee. Return to the upright position. Stretch both arms toward your right foot, bending your head down toward the right knee. Repeat 10 times to each leg.

Do not slide across from one leg to the other. Come all the

way up to a sitting position, then bend to the opposite leg. If you cannot get your head all the way down to your knee, go as far as you can without straining. Remember, you should do this exercise by arching your back.

Leg stretch #2: sit upright on the floor with your legs together, extended straight out in front of you. Point your toes. Slowly stretch forward as far as possible without hurting yourself and grasp your toes (or your ankles or calves if you cannot reach your toes). Slowly pull on the toes (or ankles or calves) and bend forward, trying to touch your forehead to your knees. Hold this position for 5 to 10 seconds, breathing normally. Sit up and repeat the process three to five times.

If you cannot get your head down to your knees, bend as far as you can. Those with rigid backs will still benefit from the stretch.

PART III

7
AN A-TO-Z OF COMMON PROBLEMS ASSOCIATED WITH EXERCISE

Most people feel good when they exercise and bad when they can't. Unfortunately, many problems can result from exercise—and then prevent you from exercising. This section will provide you with information to help you prevent injuries and other problems, so you can spend more time exercising and feeling good and less time hurting and feeling bad.

AMENORRHEA

Q *Is it true that all women who exercise eventually develop irregular periods?*

A According to various studies, from 10 to 50 percent of women who exercise heavily develop irregular periods or stop menstruating altogether. Some physicians tend to blame all irregular periods on exercise, but this is an oversimplification.

All cases of irregular menstruation require careful evaluation. They can be caused by serious conditions, such as brain tumors, hormonal disorders, infections, or any other conditions that may affect the overall functioning of the body.

Almost all cases require treatment. During a normal menstrual cycle, a woman's body produces two hormones: estrogen, which stimulates growth of tissues in the breast and the inner lining of the uterus, and progesterone, which stops this stimulation.

Some women who develop irregular periods from exercise have estrogen, but no progesterone. These women are at increased risk of developing cancer because their breasts and uterine tissues are stimulated to grow at all times. This condition can lead to uncontrolled growth, which is another name for cancer, unless these women are given replacement progesterone.

Some women lack both estrogen and progesterone. They are at increased risk of developing weak bones, which are more likely to break, and thin, dry vaginas, which are more likely to hurt during lovemaking. These women need both estrogen and progesterone replacement.

If you are a woman who exercises regularly and you develop irregular periods, don't ignore it. Check with your physician and get a complete evaluation.

ANOREXIA

Q *What is anorexia and is it true that the disease can be fatal?*

A *Anorexia* means that a person has so much self-control that he or she can stop eating. Some victims of the disease actually fast to their deaths. The condition is seen far more frequently in people who exercise than in those who don't, probably because regular exercisers are in better control of their bodies.

Interestingly, the treatment for anorexia involves stopping the anorexic from exercising. Virtually all anorexics keep their bodies in constant motion. They love to move. The most effective treatment of anorexia consists of threatening the anorexic with a ban on exercise, then rewarding the patient by lifting that ban.

Dr. Albert Stunkard, the former chairman of the psychiatry departments at Stanford University and at the University of Pennsylvania, has demonstrated that the best treatment of anorexia involves hospitalization of the patient and daily monitoring of his or her weight. Whenever the patient loses weight, he or she is confined to the room. With a weight gain, the patient is allowed free movement around the hospital. Exercise is so important to anorexics that they often resume eating just so they can exercise.

But, don't be misled. Anorexia is not a simple disease that can easily be treated by placing restrictions on exercise. It is a very complex disease, with physical and psychological complications, that can be fatal to its victims if they do not receive extensive treatment and care.

BLISTERS

Q *I am an avid jogger and I often play basketball outdoors in the summer. I love it, but I always seem to suffer from blisters. How can I avoid and/or treat them?*

A When the weather gets hot, most athletes will have to face a painful fact of summer life: blisters. They're common on hands and feet in hot weather because of the combination of heat, which increases the movement of fluid (blood serum) into damaged skin, and wetness (from perspiration), which increases friction. It's important to know the proper treatment for blisters to prevent them from getting worse and to avoid the risk of infection.

The best time to drain a blister is within two hours after developing one. Soon after a blister develops, a membrane forms around the fluid that fills the blister, delaying reattachment of the skin. Also, the sooner you treat the blister, the less fluid enters it.

To drain a blister, you'll need alcohol or some other germ-killer, adhesive tape, and a needle.

Before you drain the blister, you must clean the skin on and around it with the alcohol or another germ-killer. Then sterilize the needle. This can be done two ways: either hold the needle over a low flame for several seconds and let it cool, or soak the needle in alcohol for at least 20 minutes.

Now you're ready to drain the blister. With the sterilized needle, puncture the blister in several places near its edge, pressing down on the skin with your other hand (be certain your hands are clean) to make sure most of the fluid is released. Do not remove the top layer of skin: that will only delay healing, since it takes more than two weeks for new skin to close the wound. Removing the top layer of skin also increases your chances of getting an infection.

Once the blister is drained, tightly fasten a piece of adhesive tape over the skin. Leave it there for about four days. After that time, you can remove the tape by soaking it first so it comes off easily. Don't try to pull off the tape without wetting it first, or you might reopen the blister.

Make sure you follow this routine carefully. If you notice any signs of infection—red streaks or pus coming from the blister or severe pain—see your physician.

BLOOD IN THE URINE

Q *I recently ran my first marathon and was terrified to discover blood in my urine after the race. It cleared up on its own the next day, but it scared me. What happened and should I be worried?*

A Almost all runners have blood in their urine after running a marathon. Although exercise in itself sometimes causes blood to enter the urine, you should still see your physician for a checkup.

During hard, sustained exercise your kidneys bounce around, which sometimes causes red blood cells to leak into your urine. On rare occasions, the inner linings of an empty bladder will rub together, creating the same effect.

As a general rule, this kind of exercise-induced bleeding will completely disappear in less than 48 hours. If the blood in your urine cleared within 48 hours, chances are the bleeding was harmless and there is no cause for worry.

Nevertheless, you should have a complete medical examination to rule out other possible causes. The examination should include a urine test to check for infection, an evaluation for kidney stones, and a kidney X-ray to help rule out the possibility of a tumor.

When your doctor completes the tests and gives you a clean bill of health, you'll run with greater piece of mind.

BULIMIA

Q *What is bulimia?*

A Many athletes, especially gymnasts, long-distance

runners, and figure skaters, are very concerned about being thin. They worry about having dead weight that may slow them down or curb their competitive edge.

A preoccupation with thinness can lead to an eating disorder known as *bulimia*, which is being found in an increasing number of young, primarily female, athletes. Bulimia is related to anorexia nervosa. An anorexic refuses to eat; a bulimic, on the other hand, binges, or eats large meals, and forces herself to get rid of the food, either by regurgitation or by taking laxatives and/or diuretics. This is a routine she repeats three or four times a day. The reasons are the same: fear of being fat.

Bulimia is a secretive disorder until serious symptoms emerge. These can be a sudden drop in weight or a viral infection. If the body isn't nourished properly, its immune system suffers. Many bulimics and anorexics end up in the hospital with viral infections their weakened bodies were unable to fend off. For the athlete, these symptoms may also include a dramatic downslide in performance.

A perceptive coach can do much to persuade a bulimic athlete to seek medical help. Blood tests can pinpoint a deficiency of potassium, a mineral the body needs in large quantities. A low blood level of potassium usually does not occur in healthy individuals. But, simply replacing the potassium by taking potassium pills is not proper treatment; it does not get to the source of the problem and can delay treatment of this progressively destructive disease.

Most bulimics will deny they are vomiting or are taking laxatives or diuretics. If a physician suspects bulimia, he should order a urine check for potassium. If the urine shows increased amounts of potassium, that is good evidence the patient is vomiting frequently, since vomiting causes the kidneys to release large amounts of potassium into the urine to offset an increased blood alkalinity.

Once a bulimic is confronted with such medical evidence, she will often admit to her problem. Then she should be referred for psychological and nutritional counseling.

CALLUSES

Q *I have a thick callus just behind the ball of my foot that hurts every time I run. What can I do to treat it?*

A A callus is a thickening of the skin caused by extra pressure. Calluses are frequently caused by ill-fitting shoes. Before you attempt to treat the condition, however, you should make sure that what you have is a callus and not a wart, which looks very similar.

It is important to get the correct diagnosis because the treatment for the two conditions is quite different. Warts have deep roots that need to be removed by a physician. Calluses, however, have no roots and you can treat them yourself.

Once you're certain you have a callus, find out what caused it. First, make sure your exercise shoes fit well. If your shoes are too tight, have them stretched or get new, wider ones. If width is not the problem, check to see how your foot moves when you walk in the shoes. Your foot may be rolling inward excessively, which can cause friction. Inserting arch supports into your shoes can help to prevent that problem.

To treat the callus, soak your foot in water for a minute, then rub oil into the hardened skin. Next, gently rub the callus with an emery board or pumice stone. Be careful not to rub so hard or long that you cause bleeding.

CHAFING

Q *My fitness program is being disrupted by a simple nuisance. When I run, the skin on my inner thighs gets raw and chafed. Why does this happen, and how can I prevent it?*

AChafing results from friction, either from skin rubbing against skin or against clothing. During exercise, wetness from perspiration contributes to the problem by making the skin sticky and thereby increasing friction.

Chafing on the inner thighs has two possible causes. First, large, muscular or fat thighs may be rubbing against each other. Powdering the skin before you run can absorb some of the perspiration and reduce friction, lessening the likelihood of chafing. Second, too much material between the legs or rough stitching in that area can be abrasive to the skin. When shopping for running shorts or pants, look for those that have a minimum of material between the thighs and smooth, non-bulky seams.

CHEST PAIN

Q*I sometimes develop chest pain when I exercise in cold weather, but never in warm weather. Is this serious?*

A People with healthy hearts should not develop chest pain when they exercise in cold weather.

Your heart, in fact, works much harder in hot weather than it does in cold. More than 70 percent of the energy produced by your body is lost as heat. Less than 30 percent is used to drive your exercising muscles. When you work out, your body produces large amounts of heat. Your heart must work extremely hard pumping extra blood to bring oxygen to your muscles and also to carry heat from the muscles to your skin, where the heat can be released.

If you have a weak heart and exercise hard in hot weather, you can become overheated and suffer from heart failure. The first treatment would be to get you out of the heat and into an air-conditioned room.

If you have a healthy heart, you should have no problem exercising in cold weather. After all, your heart does not have to work as hard to cool the body. Nevertheless, a partial block in the blood vessels leading to your heart can cause a chest pain during exercise. The pain is called *angina*.

When a cold wind blows in your face, it makes your heart slow down. (This is exactly the opposite of what happens as a result of cooling your hands or feet, which cause your heart to beat faster. So, be sure to protect your extremities from the cold.) When the heart is not beating as fast, less blood is pumped to it, and people who already have a poor blood supply to their hearts could develop chest pain. Check with your doctor. The flow of blood to your heart may be partially blocked.

COLDS AND FLU

Q *Before my family and I are hit with colds or flu this season, I'd like to know if it is safe to exercise if we're still sneezing and coughing. We don't like to be inactive for too long.*

A It is usually safe for you to exercise when you have a cold provided that you do not have a fever, and your muscles do not hurt.

There is no evidence that mild exercise—walking, slow running, a few gentle laps in a pool—will make your symptoms worse or prolong recovery time. In a landmark test of military recruits suffering from infections, those who were put to bed when they became ill did not recover any faster than another group who continued with their normal training routine. Severity of symptoms and length of illness were the same in both groups.

If you have a fever or your muscles ache, you may endanger your health by exercising. During exercise, your body produces tremendous amounts of heat. This taxes your heart, which must pump blood to supply oxygen to your muscles and to your skin to dissipate your body heat. If you have a high fever before you exercise, the activity may cause your temperature to rise higher, making your heart work even harder to cool you.

Occasionally with upper respiratory infections, the heart muscle itself is affected by a condition called myocarditis, an inflammation of the muscular layer of the heart wall. Exercising with this condition can result in irregular heartbeats and even death.

Some viral infections affect your muscles, causing them to ache. Exercising while your muscles ache can cause them to tear.

If you don't have these symptoms, it is probably safe to exercise, providing you don't push yourself too hard. Expect that you will not be up to your best.

CRAMPS

Heat Cramps

Q *I play in tennis tournaments and have lost more than $100,000 over the years because I develop muscle cramps late in matches, particularly in hot weather. I have had repeated blood tests and my salt levels are always normal. What's wrong with me?*

A The most common cause of muscle cramps that occur in hot weather in athletes is dehydration. When you lose a lot of fluid, your blood volume is reduced. You may not have enough blood to circulate adequate amounts of oxygen to your muscles. Any muscle that doesn't get enough oxygen can go into spasm and hurt.

Mineral deficiencies rarely cause muscle cramps in athletes. During exercise you lose perspiration. It contains far more salt than water in relation to your bloodstream, so your blood salt level rises.

Potassium is a mineral that is found chiefly inside the cells. When muscles start to overheat, they release potassium into the veins that carry blood from the muscle. This causes the veins to widen and carry more hot blood from the muscle to the skin where the heat can be dissipated. So, blood potassium levels increase. Blood calcium levels remain the same and magnesium levels drop slightly. However, you don't lose much magnesium. The magnesium moves from the blood fluid into the red blood cells.

To prevent cramps, drink a cup of cold water before you start your match and at least every 15 minutes during the match.

Leg Cramps

Q *What causes leg cramps and how can I avoid them?*

A Leg cramps can stem from a variety of causes—from the relatively minor problem of dehydration to the more serious problem of blocked arteries. Although the pain feels the same, leg cramps should be treated differently depending on their source.

Leg cramps that occur shortly after you start exercising can be caused either by blocked arteries or, in rare cases, a mineral deficiency; leg cramps that occur after you've been exercising for an hour or more are usually the result of dehydration.

Leg cramps caused by blocked arteries and those caused by dehydration are both due to a lack of oxygen in your muscles. If you have blocked arteries, which is seen most frequently in people over 50, you will probably feel no pain while you're at rest. But, when you start to exercise your muscles need more oxygen. If your arteries are too narrow to permit the extra blood to flow into your muscles, you'll develop a muscle spasm and feel pain. If you suffer muscle cramps shortly after you start to exercise, check with your physician immediately. Blocked arteries can lead to blood clots and heart attacks.

If you develop leg cramps after you've run a long distance or have played several games of tennis, you probably just need to drink more water. When you exercise, you lose fluid at a rapid rate through perspiration. If you lose too much fluid from inside your muscle cells, you can become dehydrated, which will interfere with your normal muscle function and cause cramps. To prevent this, drink a glass of water just before you start to exercise, and a glass of water at 15-minute intervals for the duration of your exercise.

Lack of such minerals as potassium, calcium, or sodium can also cause muscle cramps after you've been exercising over an extended period of time. But this is extremely rare. If you are conscientious about drinking water when you exercise and still get leg cramps, check with your physician to find out whether you have a mineral deficiency. This could indicate a kidney or glandular problem, or may be caused by medication that can deplete certain minerals.

Leg Cramps at Night

Q *Several times I have been awakened from a sound sleep with a painful muscle cramp in my leg. Why is this?*

A You are not alone—nighttime muscle cramps strike a lot of people.

Muscle cramps during sleep are usually caused by a special muscle-tendon reflex. The word muscle comes from the Latin word for mouse. Like a mouse, a muscle has a body (the muscle) and a tail (the tendon).

When you turn over in your sleep, your muscles contract. This stretches the attached tendons. When the tendons stretch, sensitive nerve receptors send a message to your spinal cord. The message loops right back to the muscle to make it contract even more. It is an involuntary action—your thought processes are not involved. The muscle may stay contracted, resulting in a painful muscle cramp.

Treat a nighttime muscle cramp by exhausting the stretch reflex. With one hand, stretch the muscle. With the other hand, squeeze the muscle every few seconds until the cramp disappears. For example, if you have a cramp in your calf muscle, you should pull the front of your foot up with one hand to stretch the muscle. Then, squeeze the calf with the other hand.

Q *How can I prevent cramps in my calves at night?*

A Most nighttime muscle cramps can be prevented by stretching the cramp-prone muscle before going to bed. If you get cramps in your calf muscles, for instance, you should stretch those muscles by doing wall push-ups. Face a wall, standing at least four feet away. Place your palms flat on the wall, keeping your back straight. Bend your elbows so your upper body moves closer to the wall. Press your heels to the ground to stretch the calf muscles. Hold this position for a count of 10. Straighten your elbows and push up to a standing position. Repeat at least five times before you go to bed.

If stretching before bed does not prevent further cramps, check with your doctor. You may have another, less common, cause of muscle cramps, such as a blocked flow of blood to the muscle; abnormal levels of such minerals as potassium, sodium, calcium, or magnesium; a pinched nerve; or a problem with the muscle itself.

Stomach Cramps

Q *I try to wait two or three hours after eating before I exercise, but often still experience stomach cramps. Is this a normal condition?*

A Stomach cramps during exercising are common. There are two types of stomach cramps: *gaseous* and *nongaseous*. If you have cramps with gas, they are probably due to a milk intolerance; the type without gas is usually due to food remaining in your stomach when you've eaten before exercising.

To prevent nongaseous cramps, make sure your stomach is empty before you start to exercise. When food is in your stomach, your stomach muscles must continually contract to mix the food. While these muscles are working, they require a rich supply of oxygen from your bloodstream.

But, when you exercise vigorously, your other muscles require so much oxygen that your heart is unable to supply blood to both your stomach and those other muscles at the same time.

In that case, the blood supply to your stomach will be diminished and, since your stomach muscles won't get all they oxygen they need, they go into spasm, causing cramps.

You still need to keep your energy up when you exercise, especially if you participate in athletic competition. Eating three hours before you exercise should supply enough energy while lessening your chances of developing nongaseous cramps.

What you eat is also important to avoid stomach cramps. Eating a meal that is loaded with fat will markedly delay your stomach from emptying. Instead, eat mostly carbohydrates such as fruit, pasta, bread, and potatoes.

If that doesn't help, try a complete liquid meal that you can buy at a drugstore. This contains ample amounts of carbohydrates, fats, proteins, vitamins, and minerals that pass through your stomach quickly. Brand names include Ensure, Sustacal, and Nutriment.

Gaseous stomach cramps also are very common among exercisers. They are most frequently caused by a difficulty in digesting milk, so to prevent these cramps, you should stay away from milk and milk products such as yogurt, cheese, and butter.

Milk consists of an indigestible double sugar called lactose, which needs to be broken down into two digestible single sugars, *glucose* and *galactose*. Since people who get these cramps generally have a deficiency of *lactase*, the chemical that breaks down lactose, they are unable to digest milk properly.

To see if you have a lactase deficiency, avoid ingesting milk and milk products for 48 hours before you exercise. If your symptoms disappear, you should avoid them completely for eight hours before you exercise.

You may not notice any difficulty in digesting milk unless you exercise. Exercise speeds up the rate that food passes along the gastrointestinal tract, which may cause the food to pass along the intestine too fast for the lactase to work properly.

DIZZINESS

Q *I've been playing tennis for years. But, during the last year after I have served as hard as I can, I feel faint and* *dizzy and my heart beats like crazy. What causes this?*

A You probably hold your breath while you serve as do most of us. When you strain and hold your breath, your blood pressure rises tremendously.

The high blood pressure stretches your blood vessels and stimulates certain pressure sensors in the main artery that are in your neck leading from your heart. These sensors send signals back to your heart that cause it to slow down and beat with less force than usual. This response, called the carotid sinus reflex, helps lower your blood pressure.

While your heart is beating slowly, though, it is not pumping as much blood to your muscles and you develop a lack of oxygen and may become dizzy. To catch up with this oxygen debt, your heart speeds up again, beating at a much faster rate than normal until the oxygen balance is restored.

This process occurs in everyone who plays tennis—or does anything that involves straining while holding the breath— although not everyone reacts by feeling faint. The reaction you describe is unlikely to be harmful, but you should check with your physician just to be sure.

Q *For the last two years I have run regularly. Recently I have begun to suffer severe dizziness when I get up from bed after lying down. What is wrong?*

A Probably nothing, but check with your doctor anyway. The dizziness you describe often occurs in athletes, who have the slow heartbeats that are common in physically fit people. Because regular exercisers are in shape, their hearts are larger and stronger than those of out-of-shape people and can, therefore, pump more blood than usual with each beat. This means their hearts do not have to beat as often.

Dizziness often occurs when you stand up after lying down because when you stand up gravity pulls the blood away from your head. Your next heartbeat is the one that pumps blood back up to your brain. Your heart, beating slowly, does not have enough time to start its next beat to pump the blood back to your head. This lack of blood can make you feel faint, weak, and dizzy; black spots may appear in front of your eyes; and you may even pass out. This can be annoying, but it's usually not harmful.

EARACHE

Q *Is it normal to have earaches due to exercising in cold weather?*

A Many athletes complain of earaches when they exercise outdoors during cold weather. These earaches are mostly due to breathing in dry, cold air and can be minimized and often prevented.

Your inner ear produces a fluid that lubricates the mucous membranes that line the *eustachian tube*, which is the passage from your inner ear to the back of your throat. The fluid flows from your inner ear through the eustachian tube to the back of your throat. After the fluid reaches your throat, you swallow it along with your saliva.

When you exercise vigorously in cold weather, the cold, dry air you inhale can irritate the tissue lining in the back of your throat. That, in turn, can cause swelling, which can shut the opening to your eustachian tube.

Your inner ear will still produce the fluid, but, since the swelling prevents its flow through the eustachian tube, the fluid collects in your inner ear, creating pressure that can become painful.

Q *How can I prevent these cold-weather earaches?*

A There are several ways to prevent this kind of earache. First, exercise at a relaxed pace so that you don't breathe hard and fast. That way, less cold air will enter your throat. A lightweight mask that covers your mouth and nose will warm the air you breathe in.

Once the pain starts, chew some gum. The chewing motion may be enough of a stimulus to open your eustachian tube so the fluid can flow out.

You may also try a decongestant or a nasal spray. These cause body tissue to shrink and may work well enough to open the entrance to your eustachian tube.

If you have a severe problem with earaches, you probably will be better off exercising indoors with humidification where you can breathe wet, warm air instead of dry, cold air.

EYEGLASSES

Q *Whenever I exercise in the rain, the water gets on my glasses so that I can't see. And, when I exercise in cold weather, cold air condenses on them. Is there anything I can do to prevent these problems and be able to see?*

A Some simple solutions to your problem do exist.

When you run in the rain, wear a hat with a visor and keep your head down, which should keep the rain off your glasses.

When you exercise in cold weather, wear a hat—not a hood—that fits over your ears. A hood, which is usually tight-fitting, covers your face so that the water from the air you exhale will condense on your glasses and fog them up. A hat will eliminate this problem while keeping you warm.

You may also apply a defogging liquid on your eyeglasses. This liquid, available at most drugstores, contains a chemical that prevents moisture from forming on the glass.

FROSTBITE

Q *What is frostbite and how can I avoid it while working out in frigid weather?*

A Frostbite is more common than you might think, and is a particular danger for mountain climbers, cross-country skiers, and hikers—in fact, anyone who stays out in the cold for a long time, away from any easily accessible shelter.

If you know the symptoms to watch for and make sure you have access to shelter, frostbite is easily prevented no matter how cold the temperature. The Coney Island Polar Bears, a New York outdoor swimming group whose members enjoy defying the elements, go swimming on even the coldest winter days and never develop frostbite. That's because they know they can stay in the water until their skin starts to itch, burn, and turn red. Then, they get out of the water and immediately warm themselves.

When the temperature of your skin drops below freezing, ice crystals form in the fluid that is found inside and outside of your skin cells, damaging the cells. When that happens, you've got frostbite.

A set sequence of events occurs before you develop frost-bite. As your skin temperature begins to drop, your blood vessels contract, decreasing the blood flow and turning your skin white. When your skin temperature falls to 59°F, your body attempts to rewarm your skin by opening the blood vessels to increase the blood circulation to the skin's surface.

At this point, your skin will feel warm, tingly, and turn red. Once you notice these symptoms, you should immediately get out of the cold. If you stay outside, your blood vessels will again close up and your skin temperature will drop rapidly to freezing. When it reaches the freezing point, your skin will appear white and feel hard to the touch, like a frozen piece of meat.

Most of the damage from frostbite occurs during the thawing process when, as the skin warms, the skin cells may burst and be destroyed. The best way to treat frostbite and avoid any damage to your skin cells is to rewarm your extremities rapidly in water that is 100°F to 108°F. This process is extremely painful, and if the water temperature rises higher than 108°F, your skin cells may die. Make sure that you have a physician supervise this delicate treatment of frostbite to avoid complications.

HAIR CARE

Q *I shower and wash my hair in the morning before leaving the house; I also take aerobics, and shower and wash my hair in the evening. Is this harmful to my hair?*

A Vigorous exercise can go to your head. When you exercise, you will sweat. Sweat, salt, skin debris, and oil will cling to your hair.

There is nothing wrong with shampooing your hair twice a

day. You should wash your hair whenever it needs washing. Almost all shampoos on the market today are safe enough to use that often. They will not damage your hair or scalp no matter how often you use them.

Each hair shaft is covered with a protein layer called a *cuticle*. The cuticle is so tough that it will not be harmed by frequent shampooing.

Q *Are any shampoos, such as the acid-balanced type, safer or better for my hair than others?*

A Do not be misled by advertisements claiming that acid-balanced pH shampoos are safer. The cleaning agents in all shampoos are alkaline soaps and detergents. There is nothing harmful about alkaline shampoos. Some manufacturers add acids to make their products less alkaline. But, it does not change the soaps and does not make any difference to your hair. Beer, milk, herbs, and vitamins do not do much either. If your scalp is very dry, you may need to use a conditioner after you shampoo.

Q *What is the best hairstyle for my new everyday exercise class?*

A If you exercise a lot, a simple hairstyle—for men and women—will be easier to maintain. This is especially important for runners, swimmers, and other exercise enthusiasts who need to shampoo often. Choose a style suited to frequent shampooing. Hair is most manageable when it is cut to fall in its own natural way. It will make you happier because it will take less time to manage. If you must spend a lot of time curling or styling your hair after each shampoo, you may lose your interest in exercise.

HEADACHE

Q *Shortly after I finish a running race, I get a terrible headache. What causes it and can I prevent it?*

A Headaches that follow vigorous exercise are usually the result of one of two causes: a widening of the blood vessels in the brain or drinking too much water without eating after you've exercised.

During exercise, your body produces large amounts of hormones such as epinephrine, norepinephrine, and dopamine, which trigger the blood vessels in the brain to widen to permit an increased blood flow to the brain.

When the blood vessels widen they activate nerve receptors in the vessels, and this can trigger pain in some people. The headache that results is called an *effort migraine*, and is usually prevented by taking drugs like propanolol which block the hormones and prevent widening of the blood vessels.

Q *Can drinking too much water actually cause headaches after exercising?*

A Another type of headache is caused by drinking too much water after you exercise. Drinking large amounts of water—at least three glasses—dilutes the minerals in your bloodstream, creating an imbalance that causes your brain cells to swell and hurt.

Eating adds minerals which prevents this process from taking place. So, if you get very thirsty after a race, make sure to eat something along with drinking the water.

Check with your physician to make sure your headaches are not caused by any serious medical condition.

HEAT EXHAUSTION

Q *I play on my college football team. Every summer, we start two-a-day workouts. After one week, I become so weak and tired that I can't get through my workouts. What is happening to me?*

A You may have *heat exhaustion*, failure to replace the fluid that you lose during exercise. When you exercise, you lose tremendous amounts of fluid through sweating. Lack of fluid does not cause you to be thirsty. Thirst is governed by certain cells in your brain, called *osmoreceptors*. Sweat contains far less salt in comparison to blood. So, during exercise, you sweat and lose more water than salt, and the salt concentration in your blood rises continuously. The osmoreceptors in your brain won't signal that you are thirsty until you have lost between two and four pints of sweat, enough fluid to increase the salt concentration in your bloodstream sufficiently to make you feel thirsty.

Weigh yourself daily. A loss of two or more pounds may

mean that you aren't replacing all of the fluid that you lose during exercise. The treatment is to drink more fluids.

Another very common cause of tiredness in athletes is failure to replace the muscle sugar that they use up when they exercise. Many people who exercise daily go through periods of tiredness. It's usually due to lack of fluid or failure to replace muscle sugar. You replace muscle sugar by eating carbohydrate-containing foods, such as pasta, bread, fruit, pancakes, beans, and candy.

HEAT STROKE

Q *I run in the summer and often hear warnings about heat stroke. How does it occur and how can I prevent it?*

A Each year, thousands of exercisers—even professional athletes in the peak of condition—suffer from *heat stroke*, which is fainting from a sudden uncontrolled rise in body temperature during exercise in the heat. Some even die. But, this should never happen, because the body offers plenty of warnings before heat stroke occurs.

During exercise only about 30 percent of your energy is used to drive your muscles; more than 70 percent of the energy is wasted as heat. The harder you exercise, the more heat is produced. Your body does all it can to keep from overheating. Large amounts of blood are pumped from your hot muscles to your skin. Perspiration is produced and evaporates, cooling the blood as it is pumped through tiny capillaries just beneath the skin's surface.

Sometimes, however, especially when you're dehydrated, you produce far more heat than your body can eliminate, and your temperature rises uncontrollably. It is normal for your temperature to climb to around 102°F or 103°F during hard exercise, but when it rises higher than that, your muscles start to feel as if they are burning. The air you breathe in feels like it's coming from a hot furnace. Your lungs hurt and you find it very difficult to get enough air into them. You become short of breath. Your chest aches.

If this happens to you, stop exercising, get out of the sun, and immediately pour something wet over your head and shoulders. If you continue to exercise, your temperature will continue to rise. At that point, you will develop a headache and see spots in front of your eyes. You may feel dizzy and nauseous. These symptoms mean your temperature is so high that brain cells are being damaged by the heat and are losing their ability to function properly. The next step is heat stroke and loss of consciousness.

If you are not treated immediately, you can die. You can lose so much body fluid that there isn't enough left in your bloodstream to support circulation and your blood pressure will drop. You will be in shock. Your elevated blood temperature can prevent your blood from clotting, causing blood to leak from the vessels into the tissues of your brain, liver, kidneys, and heart.

The best medicine is prevention. Listen to your body as you exercise in the heat. If you detect any of the early warning signs, stop exercising and get out of the heat.

HEMORRHOIDS

Q *I have hemorrhoids that hurt so much when I run I have to stop. Is there anything I can do so I will be able to run without this pain?*

A *Hemorrhoids* are widened blood vessels in the rectum. They hurt when they fill up with blood.

You can prevent hemorrhoid pain during exercise in several ways. Take measures to soften your stools. Apply a lubricating oil to your buttocks before you run. Constipation can cause you to strain when you have a bowel movement and this, in turn, can cause hemorrhoids to enlarge. To prevent constipation, you should drink extra fluids with each meal, eat large amounts of foods containing fiber such as fruits, vegetables, and whole grains, and eat fewer foods that contain refined starch, such as white bread and sugar.

Before you start running, apply a lubricating oil such as petroleum jelly to your hemorrhoids to lessen the friction caused by the running motion.

A physician may prescribe a *glucocorticoid* (cortisonelike) cream to apply on the painful area to reduce the swelling. If that doesn't work, the next step is to get a glucocorticoid injection into the skin overlying the hemorrhoids. In severe cases, you may need surgery.

As long as you are being treated for the problem, there is no reason to curtail your running.

HYPOTHERMIA

Q *What are the effects of exercising in extremely cold weather? Can it actually lower body temperature?*

A If you dress properly, you can exercise on very cold days without being harmed. Wear several layers of relatively light loose clothing, cover your ears and fingers, and get out of the cold if your clothes become wet. Inadequate clothing or wetness can lead to *hypothermia*—below-normal temperature.

Hypothermia occurs when your body temperature has

dropped below its normal level of 98.6°F. Body temperature below 90°F can cause your heart to beat so irregularly that it may not be able to pump blood through your body.

Your body gives plenty of warning signs of hypothermia.

With a one-degree temperature drop, your speech becomes slurred and you may start to shiver. Shivering is the alternate contraction and relaxation of your muscles. It generates a lot of heat in an attempt to compensate for the heat loss.

When your temperature drops more than two degrees, you have difficulty controlling your hands. If you are skiing, for example, you may find it difficult to hold onto your poles. If this happens, seek shelter right away.

If your temperature is allowed to drop more than three degrees, you will lose control of your feet. You will stumble and may have to sit down. If you cannot use your legs to get up and get out of the cold, you are in big trouble. You need to go to a warm place immediately, or you will get even colder and can die.

One final tip—avoid going out in very cold weather after drinking alcohol. Alcohol consumption widens blood vessels near the skin, causing even more heat to be lost.

See Chapter 10 for a further discussion of exercising in hot and cold weather.

KELOIDS

Q *After knee surgery I developed a keloid. It itches and restricts my knee movement. What can I do?*

A A keloid is a very thick scar that is most common among blacks. There are several ways to effectively get rid of keloids.

Find a physician who is experienced in injecting an anti-inflammatory steroid called *triamcinolone*. Because you will need it in a very high dose, it's important that your doctor has used this drug before.

Your physician should inject the drug into the scar. This can be done as often as every third week until the scar shrinks significantly. There are side effects to this drug: the skin on your scar may become lighter, and a loss of fat underneath the scar may cause your skin to dimple. In most cases the dimpling effect is temporary, usually disappearing in less than six months. The lightening of the skin is often permanent.

If the triamcinolone injections by themselves do not work, a surgeon or dermatologist can remove your keloid surgically in a simple office procedure. About one week after the surgery, your physician should inject triamcinolone into the skin to prevent the scar from returning.

KNEE INJURIES

The careers of many top athletes, including football stars Joe Namath and Gale Sayers, have been cut short because of knee injuries. Everyone who regularly works out, either in a football stadium or a health club or by running in the neighborhood, should stop exercising when the knee hurts.

Q *I hear so much about knee injuries among well-known athletes and also people I know. Aren't there any solid, preventive measures?*

A There are two ways to prevent a knee injury or to protect an already damaged knee: wear special inserts or orthotics in your shoes and do exercises to strengthen the muscles and ligaments that surround the knee. The knee is a delicate joint that is actually nothing more than two bones held together by muscles and thick fibrous bands called ligaments.

Such exercises as leg extensions and hamstring curls also can prevent knee injuries because they thicken the ligaments and muscles in the knee joint, making them more resistant to injury.

To do leg extensions, sit on a table with a heavy weight (five pounds or more if comfortable) attached to one foot. Slowly raise and lower the leg to which the weight is attached by straightening and bending that knee. Do 10 times, rest a few seconds, and do two more sets of 10. Repeat with the other leg.

Hamstring curls also can be done with weights. Leaving the weight attached to one foot, stand on a bench with the weighted leg hanging over the side. Slowly raise the heel of the unweighted leg by bending the knee. Lower. Do three sets of 10. Repeat with other leg.

Q *I hear popping sounds in my knees when I walk or run. Is something wrong?*

A Joint sounds during exercise are harmless if you feel no pain. If it hurts when you hear the sounds, something is wrong and you should check with your doctor.

Whether or not the joint sounds are harmless depends on their origin. Bones are so soft that they can actually wear away with the least amount of rubbing. To protect your bones from this kind of wear, a tough gristle called cartilage covers the ends of bones where they come together to form a joint.

It is normal for small pieces of cartilage to break off and float in the fluid lubricating a joint. When the joint moves, the tiny pieces of cartilage may slip between the intact cartilage covering the ends of the bones and make a snapping sound. This is harmless.

On the other hand, loose pieces of cartilage may be large enough to rub against the intact cartilage and cause more pieces to break off. If this is happening, you will feel pain with the snapping sounds.

The sound could also be caused if the intact cartilage lining the ends of opposing bones rubs together. This action can damage the intact cartilage and will hurt.

If your joints make music when you exercise, but they don't hurt, keep exercising to the beat. If your joints hurt, stop exercising and see your doctor.

LIVER TESTS (ABNORMAL)

Q *I was recently hospitalized because my doctor thought I had hepatitis. One day later he sent me home and said I didn't have hepatitis. Could the fact that I am a marathon runner have anything to do with this?*

A Certainly. Vigorous exercise can release certain enzymes into your bloodstream that also appear there in large amounts when you have hepatitis or other liver disorders.

Hepatitis, or inflammation of the liver, can be caused by a virus, drugs, alcohol, or even allergies. Your liver manufactures enzymes, which start chemical reactions in your body. Under normal conditions, only very small amounts of these enzymes are released into your bloodstream. But, when your liver is damaged, it releases large amounts of these enzymes (including SGOT, SGPT, and LDH) into your bloodstream.

Many of the same enzymes are stored in your muscles and released into your bloodstream when you exercise vigorously. Routine blood tests will not tell whether the enzymes came from your liver or your muscles.

A regular exerciser who has elevated blood levels of these enzymes should stop exercising for 48 hours and be given another blood test after this time. If the enzyme level is down to normal, a diagnosis of hepatitis can usually be ruled out. If the enzyme level in the bloodstream remains high, you'll need a thorough evaluation for liver damage.

MOLLUSCUM BODIES

Q *My son is a high school wrestler. Recently, he came home with small bumps in his armpits and on his shoulders. The doctor said that they are called molluscum bodies and told us that they will go away. What should we do?*

A Take your son to a dermatologist who will treat them with a quick and easy procedure in which the small, meaty centers from each bump are scraped away.

Molluscum bodies are small bumps in the skin that are caused by a highly contagious virus. This virus can be transmitted by any skin contact with an infected person and is very common in wrestlers, since they rub against each other without protective clothing.

NOSEBLEEDS

Q *What do you do if your nose starts to bleed while you are exercising?*

A The first thing to do when your nose starts to bleed is to stop exercising. Then sit down and, while breathing through your mouth, press your thumb and first finger near the tip of your nose where the hard bone begins. Continue the pressure for about 10 minutes.

Don't lie down. This will allow the blood to drip down the back of your throat and you may swallow it, which can cause stomach cramps and possibly nausea.

More than 75 percent of nosebleeds are from the blood vessels in the lower part of your nose, so the pressure of your fingers should be enough to shut off the bleeding and allow a blood clot to form.

If you bumped your nose, check to see if it is crooked, aligned differently, moves freely, or hurts excessively—all signs that it may be broken. If you suspect that it is broken, see a physician immediately. After a few hours, the nose will be so swollen that it will be impossible to set it in its proper position.

If you get frequent nosebleeds that you know are not due to accidental bruising, you should see your physician. Nosebleeds may be a sign of high blood pressure, vitamin deficiency, nasal allergy, or clotting problems.

ODOR

Q *My wife and kids always seem to comment about my smell after I come home from jogging several miles. How can I minimize the odors?*

A Body odor is preventable. You just have to know a few simple tricks to avoid it.

Body odor that appears after exercise occurs when bacteria on your skin start breaking down fats and proteins in your perspiration. Only the sweat glands in your armpits, breasts, groin, and genital area contain fats and proteins, so body odor comes only from those areas and only when the perspiration remains on your skin long enough for the bacteria to go to work. To prevent body odor, therefore, you need to decrease the number of bacteria present on your skin.

Most soaps are not very effective in fighting odor-causing bacteria because the bacteria return to your skin just a few hours after you bathe. On the other hand, special cleansing lotions such as pHisoHex and Hibiclens, which you can get with a doctor's prescription, lower bacteria counts for a longer time.

Antiperspirants can limit odor by decreasing the amount of perspiration you produce. They cause the pores in your skin to swell shut, so the perspiration cannot get to the skin's surface to interact with the bacteria.

Another tactic is to dust your armpits and groin with a powder before you exercise. Try cornstarch, talc, or baby powder. These absorb the perspiration when it reaches your skin and can help retard the bacterial reaction.

And, always put on fresh clothes after you exercise. Unwashed clothing contains skin debris and bacteria that cause odor as soon as they become wet with perspiration.

Q *My feet smell terrible after I exercise. Is there anything I can do to prevent this?*

A Foot odor is generally caused by germs that interact with sweat and dead skin. Soap and water are the best remedies, and clean socks can prevent your shoes from smelling.

Nevertheless, if you sweat heavily, you might ask your physician if you should be treated with a special solution of 20 percent aluminum chloride—which is used in a diluted form in some deodorants—in alcohol. The solution is applied to your feet, which are then covered with Saran Wrap for several hours. The procedure can markedly decrease excessive perspiration for up to one week, but it can also irritate your skin. Furthermore, it should not be used more than once a week.

PERSPIRATION

Q *Why do I perspire more after I exercise than I do during my workout?*

A When you exercise, more than 70 percent of the energy that drives your muscles is lost as heat; less than 30 percent is used to drive your muscles. This ratio stays constant whether you exercise moderately or intensely. The harder you exercise the more heat your body produces.

Your body does everything it can to keep your temperature from rising too high. The blood vessels in your skin widen so more blood can be pumped through them, and your sweat glands are hard at work producing more perspiration. The blood flowing through the vessels in your skin is cooled by this evaporation process and returns to your organs and muscles at a lower temperature, thereby cooling the core of your body.

Your car engine works on the same principle. The engine produces a lot of heat, and water or air is pumped from the engine to a radiator to get rid of the extra heat and protect the engine.

During exercise, your heart works very hard to pump blood from your hot muscles to your skin. But, as soon as you stop exercising, your heart slows down, less blood is pumped to your skin, and your temperature rises. But, since your body is still hot and needs to be cooled, you perspire more than you did before. The same thing happens when you turn off your car engine after you drive your car. The temperature of the engine rises even though it is turned off.

Q *I am a high school basketball player. During games I perspire so much that my shirt and shorts are drenched. My teammates, who don't perspire as much, often make remarks about this. Should I do anything to stop this perspiration?*

A There is no reason to stop your body from perspiring or to be worried about your condition. You're probably in better shape than your friends are, because as your level of conditioning improves, you produce more perspiration, not less. Just make sure to drink plenty of fluids since you're losing so much in your perspiration. Drink cold water during time-outs and between periods.

Q *I am a competitive female marathon runner and I sweat heavily during exercise. I recently saw a TV advertisement for a deodorant that stated women do not sweat as much as men. Is there something wrong with me?*

A There is nothing wrong with you. Years ago it was thought incorrectly that women sweat less than men. Now we know that those studies were biased because the women tested were not as physically fit as the men.

When women reach the same level of physical conditioning as men, they sweat as much.

Thus, the expression, "men sweat while women glow," held true only before women's lib grew strong.

PLANTAR FASCIITIS

Q *During the spring and fall I jog more than usual and often find I have pain along the bottom of my heel. What causes this?*

A Pain on the bottom of the heel is a common problem both in athletes and in non-exercisers. The most frequent cause of the pain is *plantar fasciitis*, a partial or complete tear in the *plantar fascia*, the tissue that covers the muscles on the bottom of your foot.

The plantar fascia is a band of tissue that starts at your toes, runs backward along your sole, and attaches to the bone at the bottom of your heel. It acts as a support for the bottom of your foot, especially the arch. If during exercise—or even casual walking—you place enough pressure on the band to spread the toes apart or flatten the arch, you can tear the plantar fascia.

Symptoms include pain just under the *calcaneus*, the large bone at the bottom of the heel, although pain can occur anywhere along the bottom of the foot. There is usually no swelling.

Treatment for plantar fasciitis usually involves resting the foot to allow it to heal. If you participate in a sport that requires running, you'll have to participate in a nonrunning sport until you don't have any more pain. Pain is nature's warning signal, and ignoring it means risking further injury. You can continue to enjoy any sport that doesn't hurt while you do it. This usually means swimming or pulling on a rowing machine—any activity that doesn't put pressure on your foot.

If you developed this problem just from casual walking, try to restrict the amount of walking you do until you can walk without pain.

If you are recovering from plantar fasciitis put special inserts—available at most pharmacies—in your shoes to take some of the stress off the plantar fascia when you walk. When your calf muscle contracts, it stretches the plantar fascia. So, stretching your calf muscles will take some of the stress off the band and allow it to heal.

The wall push-up is a good exercise for this. To do a wall push-up, stand four feet from a wall, facing it. Put both hands flat on the wall at shoulder height. Keep your heels pressed on the ground and lean your upper body closer to the wall by bending your elbows. Hold the position for 10 seconds and relax. Do this exercise 10 times each night before you go to bed.

RUNNING INJURIES

Despite frequent warnings, many athletes and steady exercisers continue to have injuries that stem from simple wear and tear of the muscles. The average runner, for example, develops two or three serious—and unnecessary—injuries a year.

For frequent exercisers, the most common causes of avoidable injuries, which include torn hamstring muscles and Achilles tendinitis are (1) not listening to your body, and (2) not planning an exercise program that allows adequate recovery time between workouts.

Of course, you can expect to develop generalized aches and pains when you exercise and you can also expect to feel an occasional localized pain that lasts for a moment. But, if you get a localized pain that lasts more than a few seconds, your body is signaling that something is wrong. Your job is to listen.

Q *How much pain should I try to endure while exercising?*

A Once you feel pain, you should stop exercising immediately. In most cases, pain that lasts more than a second or two usually indicates that something—a tendon or muscle—is tearing, or that a bone is cracking. If you stop when you first feel the pain, you'll probably have only a minor injury that will heal in a day. If you continue to exercise with pain, you run the risk of aggravating the injury, which then could take months to heal.

Every time you exercise, your muscles are injured slightly. It usually takes 48 hours for your muscles to heal. Ideally, you should exercise vigorously every other day and rest on the off days.

If you push too hard and do more exercise than your body can handle, however, your joints, muscles, tendons, and ligaments will ache all the time. It's normal for muscles to feel a little sore as you start a workout. When you're not overtraining, your muscles and joints will feel better as you continue exercising. With overtraining, they'll feel worse as you get into your workout.

If you continue to exercise with aches and pains, you are likely to injure yourself. Stressing the body has a price: minor injuries that require extra time to heal.

To benefit most from a heavy workout, you must allow your muscles to recover before stressing them again. If muscles are stressed before they recover, they tear. That's why a good exercise regimen includes easy days. A recovery period or easy day doesn't mean you have to do nothing. Quite the contrary, you can—and probably should—still work out, but at a lower level of intensity.

Q *I took up running a year ago and I love it. It's easy and it's great exercise, but some friends say I shouldn't run every day. Is this true?*

A If you feel you want to concentrate on only one sport and you want to do that sport every day, set up your workouts to alternate hard and easy days. For example, if you run six miles a day, try alternating running six miles one day with running two miles at an easy pace on your recovery day. If you're a tennis player, you may play three hard sets on one day, then hit the ball against a wall or just volley on your recovery day.

You may also pick another sport that uses your muscles in a different way. If you run, try riding a bicycle, pulling on a rowing machine, or swimming.

Q *Is it possible to get sick from too much exercise?*

A Overtraining can cause you to develop frequent infections. Common symptoms include a sore throat, running nose, and swollen glands in your neck, armpits, and groin. Marathoner Frank Shorter reports, "When I overtrain, lymph nodes swell up in my groin." Cross-country skier Tim Caldwell says that when he overtrains, he gets colds easily.

Top athletes don't do the same hard workout every day. Neither should you.

These "rules of the game" apply to everyone, even seasoned athletes. Although people under 30 can often break the rules and still escape injury, anyone 30 and over will suffer far fewer injuries by following these rules.

Q *Can special running or jogging shoes actually help prevent injuries?*

A Many wear-and-tear running injuries are the result of the way your foot rolls after it strikes the ground. You can prevent many of these injuries by wearing the right shoes or, in some cases, orthotics, special inserts that fit into your shoes.

When you run, you land on the outside bottom of your foot and then roll inward. This rolling motion helps distribute some of the force of your foot striking the ground. The inward roll helps protect you from injury. But, as your foot rolls inward, your lower leg also twists inward, putting stress on the bottom of your foot, lower ankle, lower and upper leg, knee, and hip. If this inward roll is excessive, you run the risk of developing running injuries ranging from runner's knee to stress fractures. You'll know if it's excessive because you'll feel pain when you run.

You can limit the rolling motion in various ways. Your first solution is to wear running shoes that have a firm cup fitted around the heel. Better shoes also have a second cup outside the first to hold the inner cup—and your heel—very rigid. Good running shoes have special inserts in the sole, particularly under the inner heel and under your arch, which help prevent your foot from rolling inward excessively.

Shoes that don't have enough arch support can lead to a

variety of problems, including *plantar fasciitis*, a partial or complete tear of the fibrous sheath covering the muscles in the bottom of the foot.

Another way to prevent injury is to use special inserts to fit your foot. Most of the time you can use an inexpensive insert purchased in most running shoe stores. A custom *orthotic* is made from a cast of your foot, and looks much like an arch support. Orthotics, which are used to treat a variety of back, hip, arch, ankle, and foot problems, come either rigid (hard plastic) or flexible (soft plastic or leather). Rigid ones generally provide more foot control, while the flexible inserts are usually more comfortable.

Many athletes wear orthotics. For example, Doug Collins, former Olympic basketball star and Philadelphia 76er, wore orthotics to treat his plantar fasciitis. Ask your doctor if they might help you, too.

Runner's Knee

Q *What is runner's knee and what causes it?*

A Fifteen years ago, runner's knee was one of those sports-related problems with many treatments and no cures. A runner who developed severe knee pain would go to his doctor, and be treated with pills and rest. When that didn't help, the athlete limped to another physician, who would inject cortisone into the aching joint. That didn't work, either. A third doctor would operate. That still didn't solve the problem.

Today, we know much more about how the knee works. We also have much better ways to treat the many knee injuries runners suffer from. Studies done in 1977 by Stanley L. James, M.D., of the University of Oregon, and in 1979 by Dr.

Lloyd Smith of St. Elizabeth's Hospital in Boston, show that knee pain accounts for 30 percent of all running injuries that require more than 10 days to heal. One-fourth to one-third of these long-term problems involve the kneecap in what is commonly called runner's knee.

The back of the kneecap fits into a groove in the *femur*, the long bone of the upper leg. During running, the kneecap is supposed to move up and down as you bend and straighten your knee. If it moves sideways, it rubs against the sides of the groove in the femur and causes pain. This is called *runner's knee.*

What causes a kneecap to rub against the sides of the groove? When you run, you land on the outside bottom of your heel and roll to the inside. This natural rolling-in motion, called *pronation*, causes your lower leg to twist inward. At the same time, your kneecap may be pulled outward. This happens because your kneecap is controlled by the powerful *quadriceps*, a set of four muscles in the front of your upper leg. Three of the quadricep muscles pull the kneecap to the outside; only one pulls it to the inside, causing the kneecap to rub against the long bone of the upper leg. The greater the imbalance, the more likely it is that you will develop knee pain.

Q *Is there any treatment for runner's knee?*

A Treatment for runner's knee involves three steps, (1) stopping all running until you can run without pain, (2) strengthening the quadricep muscle that pulls the kneecap inward, and (3) wearing running shoes designed to limit pronation.

To strengthen the weak quadricep muscle, stand with your knee absolutely straight. Contract the quadricep muscles to raise your kneecap about one-half inch. Hold for a count of 10, then relax. You can do this exercise off and on all day. Your doctor may use other exercises also.

To limit pronation you should wear good running shoes. Your shoes should have the following: a rigid *counter*, the cup that goes around the heel; a strong *saddle*, the fabric running from the middle of the sole up to the lacing; a sole insert to support your arch; a flared heel that is wider at the bottom than at the top; and a strong *collar*, the padded ribbing around the opening of the shoe where it circles your ankle.

The soles of most modern running shoes already incorporate a foam insert to help limit pronation. If you need more control, try shoe inserts sold at most sporting-goods stores, or see a sportsmedicine specialist for custom inserts.

Q *How can I tell if an ache or pain I feel when I exercise is just part of my workout, or if it is really serious enough to stop exercising?*

A Many people become injured after they start an exercise program, and then decide there is something physically wrong with them that will prevent them from future exercise. That's unfortunate. The key to preventing injuries and maintaining your exercise program is to listen to your body.

It takes at least six weeks for your muscles to adapt to a new exercise program, so never push yourself when you're just starting out. Even if you feel tired after only a few minutes of exercise, obey your body's signals and stop exercising that day.

If you develop a severe pain, stop exercising immediately. On the other hand, you can probably continue exercising if you have a minor discomfort that gets better while you're working out.

Whatever your injury, don't push yourself for the sake of

putting in another mile or finishing a set of tennis. Exercise should not be painful.

Q *I run about 50 miles a week and have been injured repeatedly. Sometimes I heal very quickly; other times it may take months. What's the quickest way to recover from a running injury?*

A There is no slow or fast way to recover from a running injury. All injuries are treated by rest and rehabilitation. The amount of time you need to spend in each phase depends on how serious the injury is.

Whenever you feel pain, stop running. You'll need to rest until you can run without any pain. That can be anywhere from a few days to a few weeks and, with severe injuries, several months.

You should start rehabilitation exercises as soon as you can exercise without pain. These include jogging in place, jogging in the water (with a harness to hold you up so your feet don't touch the bottom of the pool), or bicycling, which uses many of the same muscles you use when you run. If you feel any pain while you do these exercises, stop and try them again the next day.

With all injuries, you need to listen to your body: it will let you know when your muscles are strong enough for rehabilitation exercises, then jogging and, finally, for resuming your running.

Shin Splints

Q *I've been running for several years and have been*

plagued with shin splints. What exercises can I do to eliminate the problem?

A Shin splints are usually the result of a muscle imbalance, in which the calf muscles are much stronger than the shin muscles. Calf muscles, in back of your lower leg, push the forefoot down as you run; shin muscles, in front of your lower leg, pull the forefoot up. Shin splints are felt as a generalized pain along the lateral part of the lower leg.

Preventive treatment for shin splints involves exercises to strengthen the weaker shin muscles and stretch the stronger calves.

To strengthen the shins, ride a bicycle—either moving or stationary—with toe clips that attach your foot to the pedal so you can pedal up. Do this as often and for as long as possible.

To stretch the calf muscles, do wall push-ups. Face a wall while standing at least four feet from it. Put your palms flat on the wall's surface, keeping your back straight. Bend your elbows to bring your upper body closer to the wall. Keep your heels pressed on the ground during this movement so your calves will be stretched. Hold for 10 seconds. Straighten your elbows. Repeat at least five times.

Upper Leg Pain in Runners

Q *I have been running 40 to 50 miles a week for about five years and have competed in four marathons. I have been lucky to avoid injury, except for a recurring twinge in my upper left leg. What could cause this problem?*

A Runners often develop pain in the back of their upper legs. The most common causes are: (1) a pulled or torn *hamstring muscle*, the muscle running in back of the thigh, from your buttocks to the back of your knee; or (2) a pinched nerve in the lower back, which can cause pain in the upper leg region.

How can you tell the difference? If it hurts when you squeeze the hamstring muscle and the pain stops just below the knee, the most likely diagnosis is a torn hamstring. The hamstring drives you forward when you run. The upper part of the hamstring straightens your hip while the lower part of the muscle bends the knee.

If squeezing the hamstring does not intensify the pain, and the pain you do feel extends below the knee, most likely you have a pinched nerve. When a nerve is pinched, you can feel pain anywhere along the nerve path. So, if a nerve is pinched in your lower back, you may feel pain along the nerve in back of your upper leg. It will not hurt to squeeze the muscle there because there is nothing wrong with the muscle. Also, since the muscle ends just below the knee, if the pain goes lower than that, you can be relatively sure that your problem involves a nerve, not the muscle.

If you have a pulled hamstring, you'll need special exercises to strengthen the muscle. First, however, rest until you can walk without pain. Then start exercising. Attach a light weight to the foot on your injured side. You can do this by using an ankle weight or tying a bean bag filled with sand or gravel around your foot. Stand on the other foot. Then slowly raise your heel on the weighted foot toward your buttocks by bending your knee slightly. Slowly lower your heel by straightening your knee. Repeat 10 times for one set. Rest for one minute, then do two more sets of 10.

If your pain is caused by a pinched nerve, you'll need a thorough evaluation by your physician. You may be able to continue to run, provided you do special exercises for your lower back muscles. These exercises can either change the structure of your lower back, if this is causing the pinched nerve, or strengthen the muscles to take some pressure off the nerve. Try this exercise: lie on your back with a pillow under your head. Bend your knees. With both hands, pull one knee toward your chest and hold that position for 10 seconds. Lower the leg to the floor. Repeat with the other leg. Do this exercise 25 times with each leg. Stop if you feel pain.

SKIN PROBLEMS

In our body-odor-conscious society, many people feel compelled to bathe each time they exercise. As a result, they may develop such dry and itchy skin that exercise becomes more of a burden than a pleasure.

That's a shame because bathing after each workout is unnecessary. Most of us can avoid body odor after exercising by toweling-off right away, powdering our skin to help keep it dry, and putting on fresh, clean clothes.

If you feel more comfortable washing after each time you exercise, you can do a few things to avoid irritated skin.

One trick is to take a quick shower rather than a bath. Dry skin results from a lack of moisture. Soaking in a bath strips away the protective covering that keeps the moisture in your skin. But, a quick shower is less likely to do so.

Use lukewarm water. Hot water is more likely to strip away the skin's protective covering.

So does soap—use it sparingly. The purpose of a shower is to remove old skin flakes, bacteria, sweat, and other skin secretions. Plain water can clean most of your body effectively, but you will need soap to remove bacteria-laden oil that builds up on armpits, breasts, genitals, scalp, and face.

The most important step in caring for dry skin is using a cream to lock in moisture after you shower. The effectiveness of this treatment was demonstrated in studies on calluses conducted by Dr. Harvey Blank, chairman of the Department of Dermatology at the University of Miami Medical School Dr. Blank found that soaking a dry callus in oil did not soften it. However, when the callus was soaked in water and then covered with oil while still soft, the oil prevented the moisture from evaporating, and the callus stayed soft for hours.

You can get the same effect on dry skin if you apply a moisturizing cream within 20 minutes after you shower.

SORE SHOULDERS

Q *I've noticed that when I run, my shoulders begin to ache. Do you know what is wrong?*

A Most likely, your shoulder muscles are weak, and you are straining them further by contracting them while you run. Relax your shoulder muscles and let your arms swing freely. Your hands should be held at your beltline, and your fingers should be cupped loosely. ·

To strengthen your shoulder muscles, try an exercise called a shoulder shrug. Hold a barbell in your hands, raise your shoulders for a moment, and then lower them. Perform this exercise 10 times in a row.

Nevertheless, shoulder pain might signal some other problem. So, it is best to check with your physician before attempting to strengthen your shoulder muscles.

STRESS FRACTURES

Q *About a month ago, I started to feel a pain in my left foot. It started as a slight pain when I ran. When I stopped, the pain went away. As I continued my daily exercise, the* *pain returned and got increasingly worse. What is wrong with my foot and how can I get rid of this nagging condition?*

AYou may have a *stress fracture* in your foot, a small, surface bone crack caused by the repeated trauma of exercise. When you run, your foot hits the ground with a force equal to about three times your body weight. This force is transmitted to your feet, legs, and pelvis. During long-distance running, the foot can hit the ground more than 5,000 times a mile. It's easy to see how a repeated stong force on your bones can cause a crack.

With the current popularity of fitness activities, doctors are seeing more and more exercise-induced stress fractures. Common sites are the front of the feet, the lower leg, upper leg, and pelvis.

If you get a pain in any area that hurts more every time you exercise, stop exercising and check with your doctor. Continued exercise will extend the injury.

A simple "finger" test helps diagnose a stress fracture. Usually, a stress fracture will hurt when you press on it with your finger both from above and below the site. An injured tendon or ligament, on the other hand, will usually hurt only when pressure is applied from one side. Unfortunately, X-rays are usually not sensitive enough to detect the tiny crack of a stress fracture.

The best treatment for a stress fracture is rest. If you don't rest, you can extend the crack all the way through the bone. Four to six weeks of rest are usually enough to allow healing. Casts rarely are necessary.

You can keep fit while your stress fracture heals by doing exercises that will not put stress on the injured bone. For example, you can ride a bicycle or swim while your injury heals.

We don't know why some people are more prone to develop

stress fractures than others. Interestingly, we do see them more often in people who don't drink milk and also in those who start an exercise program after a long period of inactivity. Women who don't menstruate are also more likely to develop stress fractures, because they often lack *estrogen*, the feminizing hormone that helps to keep bones strong.

TOENAILS

Q *When I was training for my first marathon last year, one of my toenails turned black, and fell off. What's the cure?*

A Athletes in almost every sport can develop a common painful injury known as *black toenail.*

Black toenail is usually the result of old blood collecting under the nail. It is usually due to shoes that are too short or too wide. Either way, your toes rub against the front part of the shoe, raising the toenail and causing the tiny blood vessels under the nail to break and leak blood. The red blood cells release a pigment that forms a black-and-blue spot under the nail.

If the nail doesn't hurt, no treatment is required. If it hurts when you run, put tape over the nail to hold it in place. In several weeks, your nail will grow out and attach to its bed. Nevertheless, replace your ill-fitting shoes with shoes that fit so that you won't develop the same injury again.

If the black toenail is very painful, check with a physician. Usually he will treat the injury by making a small hole in the center of the nail to drain the collected blood. This is a simple procedure done in the office.

Black toenail can also be caused by a fungus. If you have a fungus, your doctor can treat it with antifungus pills.

VARICOSE VEINS

Q *Can wearing support hose during exercise prevent varicose veins?*

A No, and they won't even keep varicose veins from enlarging during exercise. Normally, valves in the veins in your legs help to keep the blood flowing in one direction only. If the valves do not close properly, the blood is allowed to back up and collect in the veins, causing them to swell up and form large blue lines on the legs, called varicose veins.

Support hose wrap around the legs and are supposed to compress the veins so that they won't swell up. They do this job well when you sit or lie down. However, when you exercise, you don't need support hose.

During exercise, you alternately relax and contract your muscles. When you relax your muscles, the veins near them fill up with blood. When you contract your muscles, they squeeze and compress the veins near them, forcing the blood out of the veins toward your heart. The force of the contracting muscles is so great that the additional force exerted by the support hose is insignificant by comparison.

Support hose can tire you during exercise by reducing heat loss and causing body temperature to rise.

Q *I've noticed that many professional athletes have large, blue veins in their arms and legs. Are these varicose veins? Is this proof that heavy exercise can cause varicose veins?*

A No, on both counts. Exercise can help prevent varicose veins. It does not cause them. The veins are located in a fat pad underneath skin and over muscles. Athletes have little fat, so their veins are closer to and more prominent in the skin.

VOMITING

Q *I am a 25-year-old female distance runner. During the finishing sprint of a hard race, I often develop severe stomach pains and then vomit. Afterward, I have a sore throat and a sour taste in my mouth. What is wrong?*

A It sounds as if your stomach produces too much acid.

Stomach linings normally produce acid that helps break down food so it can be absorbed into the bloodstream. During vigorous exercise, the stomach produces increased amounts of acid. This acid can irritate the stomach lining and cause vomiting. Once in your mouth, the acid can cause a sore throat and a sour taste.

Try taking antacids 20 minutes before you race. They can be bought without a prescription at any drugstore. Avoid carbonated and caffeinated drinks. If that doesn't work, ask your physician to prescribe *cimitidine*, a medication that decreases stomach acid.

8
EXERCISE AND DISEASE

ARTHRITIS

Q *I am approaching 60 years of age and my doctor has recently informed me that I am beginning to have arthritis. Can exercise help me to deal with this disease?*

A Exercise can help people who suffer from arthritis, an inflammation of the joints that afflicts more than 75 million Americans. However, because they could increase their pain by putting too much strain on their joints, arthritis sufferers should choose their exercise carefully.

Arthritis is often very painful, leading sufferers to shun exercise. But, one key to treating arthritis is to prevent movable joints from stiffening. The way to prevent that is by exercising.

Exercise brings oxygen to *cartilage*, the white gristle that lines the end of bones where they form joints. There are no blood vessels in cartilage, so it gets its oxygen from fluid that bathes the joint. Every time you put pressure on a joint, the fluid is forced out of the sac that encases it, bringing fresh oxygen to the cartilage. When you relax the joint, the fluid returns to the sac. The cartilage needs this fresh supply of oxygen to keep from getting brittle.

However, the cartilage in most people with arthritis is extremely fragile and, if too much force is applied to joints, the cartilage can break, thus preventing joints from moving freely.

Running or jogging, for example, should be avoided, because you land with three times your body weight, putting great stress on the joints. Also avoid sports that require frequent jumping, such as basketball or soccer.

Swimming, walking, and riding a stationary bicycle are all good sports for people with arthritis. Swimming is safe because the buoyancy of the water supports your body, thereby limiting the force on your joints. Walking is also good because you're never completely off the ground when you walk. And riding a stationary bicycle is safe, too, because pedaling puts little pressure on your joints, and you have less chance of falling and breaking a bone than when riding a moving bicycle.

Q *I have been running for many years. Recently, I heard that running causes arthritis. Is this true?*

A No sport will cause arthritis unless it hurts when you do it. A recent study from Boston Children's Hospital showed that long-time runners are no more susceptible to developing joint pains than swimmers. This is very reassuring because the water cushions the joints of swimmers and prevents them from being exposed to great forces.

Q *My aunt has been bedridden for two months and, although she is improved, she is too weak to walk and has become arthritic. What exercises can she do to help regain her strength?*

A Since your aunt is very weak, it is safest if she exercises in water, which alleviates the pressure that exercise usually puts on your muscles and joints. When you are immersed in water up to your neck, the buoyancy lifts you up so you need to support only one-tenth of your body weight.

If your aunt can stand, she might try walking across a swimming pool as many times as she can until she feels tired. She could also try doing calisthenics in the water.

If she is too weak to stand, have her sit in a pool immersed to her shoulders. To exercise her arms, she can move a light sponge ball back and forth. To exercise her legs, she should raise and lower each leg until she feels tired.

If you want to help in devising an exercise program for your aunt, contact your local YWCA or YWHA, which often have water exercise programs. And, if you want to learn more about water exercises, write to the President's Council on Physical Fitness and Sports, Washington, D.C. 20201 and ask for their free pamphlet on aqua dynamics.

CRUTCHES

Q *A few weeks ago I broke my leg and have been using crutches ever since. Before I was injured I ran about 70 miles a week. Now, walking just a short distance exhausts me. Could I have lost my conditioning so quickly?*

A More likely, walking with crutches is exhausting you.

You now rely on your arms to propel you and carry most of your weight. Your arms are naturally weaker than your legs because they have not been exercised as heavily as your legs were during running.

Your heart must now work harder to pump blood to your arms than it does to pump blood to your legs because the blood vessels in your arms are small and offer greater resistance against the flow of blood.

DIABETES

Q *At the age of 47 I began to develop diabetes. Is it true that exercise can help me avoid taking insulin?*

A Most people who develop diabetes after 40 can control their blood-sugar level without taking insulin. They can do this by keeping their weight at normal levels, eating less fatty food and more fiber-containing food, and exercising regularly.

Insulin, a chemical that is produced by your pancreas, moves sugar from your bloodstream into your muscles, liver, and other tissues. People who develop diabetes early in life often have little or no insulin in their bodies. But, most people who develop diabetes after age 40 do have some insulin. They develop high blood-sugar levels because their cells don't use the insulin properly, and sugar remains in their bloodstream rather than entering their tissues.

In order for sugar to enter cells, the cells must have enough insulin receptors on their membranes. Insulin cannot push sugar into the cells until it has bound the insulin receptor on the cell. Anything that reduces the number of these receptors on the cell membranes will make your cells less responsive to insulin.

Being overweight reduces the number of insulin receptors.

When your fat cells are full, the receptors fold inside the cells; when they are empty, the receptors move outside the cells so they can bind the insulin more easily to them. So, the less fat you have, the more your body can use your natural insulin.

For this reason, you should also avoid fatty foods, which also reduce insulin receptors.

And exercise is one of the best ways to control diabetes, because it helps increase the number of insulin receptors also.

Even if you follow these suggestions, do not stop taking insulin without checking with your physician. Only he will know if watching your weight, dieting, and following a regular exercise program can control your diabetes enough for you to stop taking insulin.

Q *I am a diabetic. What precautions should I take before I exercise?*

A Check your urine for the presence of *ketones*, breakdown products of fat metabolism that accumulate in the bloodstream and then pass into the urine. Ketones form because the body cannot utilize sugar properly and, therefore, uses too much fat. Exercising with ketones in the bloodstream can cause nausea, muscle weakness, headaches, and severe stomachaches.

Checking for the presence of ketones is easy. Dip a testing paper called Ketostix (available without a prescription in any pharmacy) into the urine. If the paper turns purple within a few seconds, ketones are present and you should not exercise. If the urine is free of ketones, however, exercise can be safely included in the day's activities.

On rare occasions, a ketone-free diabetic may develop a low

blood-sugar level during a workout. Several signs indicate its onset: developing a rapid heartbeat, breaking out in a cold sweat, becoming shaky all over, or feeling very hungry. If any of these symptoms appear, immediately drink something with sugar in it, such as orange juice or Coca-Cola. This will raise your blood sugar level almost instantly and bring you back to normal. Nevertheless, you should not exercise for the rest of the day.

EPILEPSY

Q *I am an epileptic who was never encouraged to exercise. Is exercise safe for me? I would like to begin a program and I'm not sure what sport to choose.*

A In 1978, Patty Wilson, a 17-year-old epileptic, ran from Minnesota to Washington, D.C., a distance of 2,000 miles. Her run was sponsored by the Epilepsy Foundation of America to demonstrate how much physical exertion epileptics can undergo.

People who suffer from epilepsy, a condition that affects approximately 2 million Americans, should be encouraged to live full lives, which include exercise. With a few exceptions, most epileptics should be able to participate in a variety of exercises.

Epilepsy is a disorder in which the electrical rhythms of the brain are disturbed, causing fainting, unconsciousness, or involuntary movement (seizures). During a seizure, an epileptic becomes disoriented and afterward his responses are often dulled. Therefore, an epileptic should not participate in any sport that could leave him in a precarious position, such as diving, long-distance swimming, parachute jumping, and horseback riding.

Many people incorrectly believe that vigorous exercise will

cause seizures because such exercise can lower oxygen levels in the brain and interfere with normal brain function. In fact, it is extremely rare for seizures to be caused by exercise. With their doctor's approval, most epileptics can run marathons, play football, and participate in many other vigorous sports.

HEART ATTACKS

Q *I have suffered a heart attack. My doctor says I'm completely recovered and ready to resume exercising. I want to remain healthy. Is it safe to exercise?*

A Although you may be afraid of exercising after you've had a heart attack, you should know that exercise can reduce your chances of getting a second heart attack. It can also help you lose weight, increase your endurance, elevate your mood and, most important, help you to resume a normal lifestyle.

Years ago, doctors told patients that once plaques formed in their arteries, they were there forever. They believed that one heart attack necessarily led to another. Heart-attack victims were usually sent to bed to die, and they usually did.

Now there is evidence that plaques can be dissolved and reabsorbed back into your bloodstream if you lower your blood-cholesterol level to less than 160 milligrams. The average level for Americans is about 150 to 300 milligrams. Losing weight will help lower your blood-cholesterol level, and weight loss is activated by exercise.

What kind of an exercise program should you start, and how should you start it?

First, check with your doctor. Most likely you will take an exercise electrocardiogram. Most physicians order this test three weeks after the patient has had a heart attack. The test can predict how much exercise a patient's heart can tolerate.

The rules for training the heart of a person who has had a

heart attack are the same as for someone who has not had one. The only difference is that it may take longer for the heart attack victim to reach the goal of exercising vigorously enough to raise his or her pulse to about 100 beats a minute for 30 minutes three times a week.

It is extremely important to have closer supervision than usual for your first exercise sessions. Follow the same precautions recommended in the previous section for people who have high blood pressure. Usually you start by alternating jogging and walking for 10 minutes. If you feel pain or get too tired, stop. You should perform this routine three times a week, never on successive days.

Your progress should be an individual affair and depend on how you feel. Make sure you don't add more than five minutes of exercise each week.

If you feel any of the following symptoms while you're exercising, stop and check with your physician as soon as possible: chest tightness or pain, lack of muscle coordination, shortness of breath, irregular heartbeats, fainting, tiredness, lightheadedness, dizziness, or excessive muscle soreness.

The following symptoms after exercise may mean you've done too much: inability to sleep at night, extreme fatigue, muscle soreness, nausea, or muscle cramps.

The speed of your return to your regular activity will depend on your progress and on the amount of damage your heart attack did to your heart.

HIGH BLOOD PRESSURE

Q *I swim and take regular exercise classes. What is the best treatment for my high blood pressure while maintaining an exercise program?*

A Many of the more than 35 million Americans who have high blood pressure take medication to help protect them from developing a heart attack or stroke. While medications to treat high blood pressure can help regular exercisers continue their fitness program, some sports may still be quite dangerous for people with this condition.

The best medications to treat high blood pressure in regular exercisers are clondine (brand name Catapres), methyldopa (Aldomet), and prazosin (Minipress). All of these prescription medications do not affect heart or muscle function during exercise. Beta blockers such as propranolol (Inderal), on the other hand, cause muscle tiredness and weakness and may limit the amount of exercise you can do. Diuretics dehydrate you and reduce your endurance. If you do take the potassium-wasting kind, make sure to take potassium supplements because diuretics drain your body of potassium, which is needed to prevent you from tiring and developing muscle injuries during exercise.

If you have high blood pressure, check with your doctor for the best course of treatment. This usually consists of regular exercise, cutting back on salt intake, increasing calcium intake, losing weight if you're overweight, and stopping the use and consumption of all stimulants such as tobacco, coffee, tea, chocolate, and caffeine-containing soft drinks. If these steps don't work to reduce your high blood pressure, your doctor will most likely prescribe medication.

If you use exercise with other methods of lowering your blood pressure, be very careful about participating in sports that require you to hold your breath when you contract your muscles. Many high-blood pressure patients have aggravated their condition by serving hard in tennis. Also, weight lifting and swimming underwater for more than 10 seconds should be avoided.

Holding your breath when you contract your muscles causes the pressure in your blood vessels to rise to very high levels. A person with a normal blood pressure of 120/80 can have his or her blood pressure rise to 300/240 while lifting weights; so, you can imagine its impact on someone with preexisting, high blood pressure.

Start-and-stop exercises can be dangerous; a sudden burst of energy can cause irregular heartbeats. Under proper medical supervision, walking, jogging, swimming, cycling, and dancing are all good exercises for heart patients.

Q *I am 60 years old and have been taking diuretics for several years to treat my high blood pressure. I frequently become very weak and tired. My doctor says I'm low on potassium and wants me to take potassium pills, but I heard they are dangerous. Can't I get potassium from eating bananas and meat?*

A For high blood pressure, doctors commonly prescribe diuretics, each of which can cause you to lose up to 1,000 milligrams of potassium per day. Although you can make up the lost potassium by eating bananas and meat, some potential problems make these sources less than effective.

To make up for the potassium lost through taking two diuretics a day, you would have to eat between 5 and 10 bananas a day. This would add up to 600 extra calories daily, which could aggravate your high blood pressure by adding extra fat to your body. Meat is also a good source of potassium, but it is also loaded with sodium (salt), which raises blood pressure.

Some diuretics cause less potassium loss than others. However, these diuretics, such as dyrenium, spironolactone, and amiloride, often are less effective in eliminating sodium from your body. Ask your doctor if you may substitute them for the ones you are currently taking.

SURGERY

Q *Can exercise be used to speed my recovery from upcoming surgery?*

A Exercising both before and after an operation can speed your recovery and help you return to your normal daily routines a lot faster.

After an operation, it will be a while before you can use the part of your body where the surgery took place without feeling pain. People who are physically strong are able to compensate for the disability of one muscle or muscle area by using stronger muscles in the surrounding area. This allows the healing area to recover and regain strength.

For example, an operation on your thumb may make it difficult to perform such simple tasks as opening a jar. But, if you've developed strong upper arm muscles before the operation, you'd be able to use the force of those muscles to perform the task. If those muscles are weak, however, you'd need to use your thumb, subjecting it to more pain and possibly delaying the healing process.

An exercise program after an operation will also help you recover faster. When tennis star Billy Jean King underwent successful knee surgery a few years ago, she was soon back on the courts. Her rehabilitation was relatively short because she exercised and strengthened the muscles supporting the knee. That way, the healing joint was aided by other, stronger muscles so it was not overly stressed during her recuperation.

Here's a hint for anyone anticipating knee, foot, or leg surgery: strengthen your arm and chest muscles before the operation. You'll find it easier to manage on crutches.

You strengthen a muscle by exercising it against resistance. Do this by lifting a weight 10 times, rest for a minute, and then do two more sets of 10 lifts, resting between each set. To strengthen your arms, do the weight lifts while standing. To strengthen your chest muscles, do *bench presses*—lie on the floor lifting the weights with your arms. Do these exercises every other day. Start with weights under five pounds. As you become stronger, gradually increase the weights.

ULCERS

Q *Can exercise help me to prevent my ulcers from recurring?*

A There is both good news and bad news about ulcers. The bad news is that although ulcers were once considered a disease of workaholic executives, they are being found increasingly in every segment of the population. In fact, ulcers plague one out of every 20 Americans.

"Ulcers are no longer the disease of the upper-echelon—executives and managers," says Dr. Ronald E. Costin, medical director of Eastern operations for the Life Extension Institute, which gives thousands of medical exams each year. "They now occur most frequently among foremen and lower-level supervisory employees. Also, we're seeing more ulcers among young people. Even among adolescents, it's a significant trend."

The good news is that with proper treatment, including regular exercise, even the most painful ulcers can be controlled.

Stomach and upper-intestinal ulcers are associated with a marked increase in stomach acidity. This hyperacidity, combined with other stomach chemicals such as *pepsin* (an enzyme that begins the digestion of proteins), can cause a break in the mucous membrane lining of your stomach or the upper part of your small intestine. When this happens, various symptoms will occur. These include a burning in the middle or left side of your stomach that disappears when you eat, a sour taste in your mouth, a white coating on your tongue, burning in the back of your throat, and burping.

If you have any of these symptoms, check with your doctor to determine if they are being caused by an ulcer or some other stomach irritation. If you have an ulcer, your doctor will probably tell you to stop drinking alcohol, coffee, tea, chocolate drinks, and any soft drinks containing caffeine, all of which increase the acidity in your body. Tobacco does this as well.

Your doctor may also prescribe medication to decrease your acidity and recommend exercise. Why exercise?

Stress and tension increase the amount of acid in your stomach. And physical activity—especially if it's not competitive—is an excellent tension-reducer. So, a simple, enjoyable way to fight stress, reduce acidity, and control your ulcer is to do regular exercise. Any continuous exercise will do.

WHEELCHAIR-BOUND

Q *Is there any way for those of us who are wheelchair-bound to participate in the fitness boom?*

A Being in a wheelchair is no reason not to be physically fit. You can effectively get your pulse rate up to 100 beats a minute—which is what you need to stengthen your heart—by exercising your ams continuously for at least 10 minutes.

One of the easiest ways to exercise your arms is to push the wheels of your wheelchair. If you do this indoors, you'll need an extra-wide treadmill to keep your wheelchair from moving. The treadmill will probably have to be custom-made, since it is a special item that isn't usually sold in sporting-goods stores. If you are doing this exercise outdoors, make sure you stay on level ground, since you don't want to lose control of your wheelchair.

Either way, follow the rules for heart stengthening. Start your exercise program by exercising until your arms hurt or feel heavy. Then stop and wait 48 hours before exercising again.

There are two other effective methods for exercising your arms; one is using arm pulleys, the other, punching a speed bag. Arm pulleys may be purchased in most sporting-goods stores, and cost anywhere from $150 to $600 depending on the quality of the materials used. Two basic types are available. One attaches to the wall. The other has a pulley that attaches to a pole so you don't need to drill holes in your walls. An arm pulley consists of two weights that rest on the floor, shoulder-width apart, and a rope that comes up from the weights and loops through the pulley. The weights are detachable, so as your arms get stronger, you can progressively add heavier weights.

The task is to pull the rope toward you over the pulley, lifting the weights as high as you can. You should start with a weight that you can lift easily. For some people, that may be as little as one or two pounds. You should pull on the rope slowly and continuously, gradually working up to 10 minutes. When you are comfortable doing this, try working up to 30 continuous minutes, which is all you need for maximum heart strengthening. Once you've worked up to 30 minutes of exercise, you can gradually start increasing the weights.

Punching a speed bag for at least 10 minutes is an equally effective arm exercise. A speed bag is a light punching bag used by boxers during training. You can buy one in most sporting-goods stores for between $40 and $300, depending on the quality of materials. They are often available on telescopic poles, which may be adjusted to any height.

Punching a speed bag is not complicated. Just make sure you position yourself close enough to the bag to reach it easily, but far enough away to keep the bag from hitting you in the face when it rebounds. If you wish, you may protect your hands by wrapping tape around your knuckles or wearing gloves.

Probably the simplest exercise is conducting an imaginary orchestra while seated. By moving your arms vigorously in the air while listening to music, you can increase blood circulation and train your heart. For maximum benefit, you should "conduct" 30 minutes every other day.

9
ALCOHOL, DRUGS, AND EXERCISE

ALCOHOL

It may be surprising to you to find that many athletes believe alcohol helps their athletic performance. It does not. The prestigious American College of Sportsmedicine declared that alcohol taken before or during exercise will not improve athletic performance and may, in fact, retard it.

Alcohol depresses the activity of your central nervous system, making you slower, tiring you sooner, and dulling your thought processes.

Alcohol tires you more quickly than usual for several reasons. First, alcohol decreases the force of your heart's normal contraction and increases its oxygen needs so your cardiovascular system must work harder. Second, it decreases the flow of blood to your muscles and interferes with their ability to burn fat for fuel.

You perspire more when you drink alcohol. This perspiration robs you of the fluid you need to keep your body going, especially during hard exercise such as running a race or playing soccer, tennis, or handball. If you lose enough fluid, you can become dehydrated and, therefore, tire earlier.

Alcohol also dulls your senses. It impairs eye/hand coordination, accuracy, and balance—all of which are very important if you're skiing, skating, or playing basketball, hockey, or a racquet sport.

Having alcohol in your bloodstream during exercise in cold weather can be extremely dangerous because it numbs the senses. A person who has been drinking isn't as sensitive to pain and may not notice the twinges and burning sensations that are the early signs of frostbite. Without feeling these sensations, a person might not get indoors in time to prevent severe skin or tissue damage.

With a list of negatives this long, and warnings from leading sportsmedicine experts that exercise and alcohol don't mix, why do some athletes contend that alcohol rejuvenates them and makes them faster? Most likely it's because the alcohol makes them think they are doing a better job than they really are.

Q *I am an alcoholic enrolled in a program to stop drinking. Can a regular exercise program help me lick alcoholism?*

A Exercise can play a major role in the treatment of alcoholism, but it may be exceedingly dangerous if your heart has been damaged by drinking.

When you exercise, your mood is often elevated and this good feeling, which may last 6 to 18 hours, can counteract the depression that often accompanies withdrawal from alcohol. A regular exercise program can also help alcoholics, who often are in poor physical condition, improve their fitness, lose weight if necessary, and strengthen their hearts.

But, check with your physician before starting such a program. Alcohol can damage the heart muscle, and many chronic alcoholics over the age of 40 have weak hearts that cannot pump the extra blood their bodies need during vigorous activity. If your heart is weak, you might pass out or even suffer a heart attack while exercising.

Q *Why does eating something while drinking alcohol help prevent a person from becoming drunk?*

A You are technically drunk when your blood-alcohol level reaches five parts per thousand. Two factors influence whether or not you reach that point: how rapidly the alcohol gets into your bloodstream and how rapidly your liver breaks it down.

Your liver breaks down alcohol at the rate of one-third of an ounce per hour. That translates into about 12 ounces of beer, 5 ounces of wine, or a half-jigger of hard liquor. You can't change the rate at which your liver breaks down the alcohol you consume, but there are several things you can do to slow its absorption into your bloodstream before it reaches your liver.

Anything you can do to keep the alcohol in your stomach longer will delay its entry into your bloodstream. Even a small amount of food in your stomach keeps the alcohol there longer and delays its absorption. So, before you drink, eat—preferably foods containing fat, such as whole milk, cheeses, fatty meats, or buttered toast. Fats keep food in your stomach significantly longer than any other kind of food.

Also, the more you dilute alcohol, the slower the absorption rate and the slower the rise in blood-alcohol levels. You can dilute alcohol by mixing it with other fluids such as water, tonic, ginger ale, or juice.

And, learn to drink slowly. By introducing alcohol into the liver slowly, you give that organ more time to break down the alcohol and prevent your blood-alcohol level from rising too high.

One more precaution: remember to drink in moderation.

Q *What is the safest way to sober up a drunk person?*

A Rest is the best, safest remedy. An intoxicated person also should drink extra, nonalcoholic fluid, because alcohol dehydrates the body. Dehydration is one of the causes of hangovers. Plain water or fruit juices are best.

Recovery time depends on several factors, including the amount of alcohol consumed. You can do nothing to increase the rate at which your liver breaks down the alcohol circulating in your blood. The liver processes alcohol at a fixed rate that works out to about 12 ounces of beer per hour, 5 ounces of wine per hour, and two-thirds of a jigger of hard liquor per hour.

A cold shower, rather than sobering up an intoxicated person, could kill him. The sudden shock may cause the person's blood pressure to rise. If the person already has high blood pressure or a weak heart, a blood vessel could burst, causing a stroke, or the heart could start to beat irregularly, causing a heart attack.

Coffee has no sobering effect. The caffeine in coffee is a stimulant that will only turn the person into a wide-awake drunk. It will not improve his or her ability to think, reason, or react.

Exercise, such as walking around the block, may damage the person's brain. Intoxication is often associated with low levels of blood sugar. Walking may deplete the body's already meager sugar reserves. A drunk person could develop a very low blood-sugar level, which could then lead to brain damage.

AMPHETAMINES

Q *I read recently that some professional baseball players take amphetamines (greenies, beanies, and uppers) to help them play better. Do these pills really help?*

A Taking amphetamines will not improve strength, speed, coordination, or endurance. They may increase your concentration, however, which in the case of a batter, would enable him to block out the sounds of a crowd while he concentrates on the pitcher.

Taking amphetamines can interfere with your judgment, though. In the book, *Ball Four*, baseball pitcher Jim Bouton describes a fellow pitcher who, after taking amphetamines, refused to be taken out of the game. He insisted he was pitching very well, although he had just thrown three, consecutive homerun balls.

In football, 150-pound halfbacks on amphetamines, have been known to try to knock down a 300-pound tackle through a hole in a line.

Furthermore, amphetamines make you less responsive to pain, the body's protective mechanism. Bicyclist Tom Simpson, at the time one of the best bike racers in the world, died of heat stroke while on amphetamines in the 1967 Tour de

France. The amphetamines allowed him to ignore the pain and other warning signals of heat exhaustion, so he rode on to his death.

ANABOLIC STEROIDS

Q *What is the purpose of taking steroids and how do they improve athletic performance?*

A The body produces anabolic steroids in small amounts. Some physicians believe these hormones help to heal damaged tissue. In the past, artificial steroids were given to people who couldn't produce their own because of disease, malnutrition, severe weight loss, or severe burns. In recent years, however, many male and female athletes—especially weight lifters, shot-putters, and discus throwers—have been taking large doses of anabolic steroids by pill or injection in the belief that the synthetic hormones will give them stronger and larger muscles.

Anabolic steroids do, in fact, seem to help some athletes recover faster from their workouts, but only those already doing rigorous strength training. This potential benefit is still being debated by scientists. The steroids will not help a novice weight lifter or a high school wrestler to gain strength. This difference is due to the fact that athletes not already working at their maximum won't benefit from the faster recovery time—their workouts are not sufficiently severe to prevent them from working out for several days at a time. The extra work allowed by the faster recovery is what makes the world-class athletes stronger.

But, more importantly, artificial male hormones in large doses are unsafe. Liver cancer, hepatitis, and heart attacks have been reported in young athletes taking these hormones. In addition, they prevent the body from making its own male hormones in both men and women. In males, this can cause sterility; in females, it can cause irregular menstrual cycles and masculinization—including male fat distribution, large muscles, and hair all over the body.

Anabolic steroids can also cause acne, headaches, high blood pressure, increased levels of fat in the bloodstream, and a manic state in which the athlete thinks he or she can do more than he or she really can.

In all, anabolic steroids have more potential risks than benefits.

ANTIBIOTICS

Q *I am a competitive marathon runner. If I develop an infection, such as a virus, when I am about to run an important race, should I take antibiotics just before the competition?*

A You can safely take antibiotics before a race. There is no evidence whatsoever that antibiotics such as ampicillin, penicillin, or tetracycline interfere with strength, speed, endurance, or coordination.

ANTIHISTAMINES

Q *Will taking cold pills before I run a race help ease a stuffy, running nose?*

A Taking decongestants and antihistamines when you have a cold can be counterproductive when you are exercising.

These medications will shrink the swelling in your nose and decrease some of your nasal secretions. Most people breathe through their mouth, not their nose, when they work out vigorously. (The openings in your nose are too small to permit enough air to be taken in during hard exercise, even if you don't have a cold.) So, shrinking the swelling in your nose won't have much impact during exercise.

Taking cold medicines that stop a running nose by curtailing mucus formation can make breathing harder during exercise. Mucus helps moisten the linings to your air passages; clean bacteria, cell debris, and germs from your air passages; and makes breathing easier. So, you want your nose to run when you exercise.

Many cold preparations on the market today make you produce less saliva and respiratory mucus. Your throat may feel dry and your nose may burn and itch. The dryer, thicker secretions that accumulate can block the flow of air into your lungs.

Antihistamines make many people feel drowsy. If you take them before you exercise, you may feel tired enough to cut your workout short.

ASPIRIN

Q *Does aspirin work to relieve the aches and pains of exercise and is it safe?*

A Aspirin has been used as a pain-killer for nearly 100 years. In that time, billions of aspirin tablets have been taken by millions of people to relieve everything from toothaches to arthritis. Many athletes use aspirin to relieve muscle soreness after a hard exercise workout.

Each time you exercise vigorously, your muscles are slightly injured. Muscle cells respond by producing hormone-like substances called *prostaglandins*, which cause muscle inflammation and soreness. Aspirin helps to prevent the formation of these pain-inducing hormones, and, in turn, prevent and relieve the muscle aches and tightness you feel during exercise.

Despite its effectiveness and widespread use, aspirin can be dangerous for some people. Aspirin causes the mucuos lining of your stomach to produce large amounts of acid that, in some instances, results in nausea, vomiting, pain, belching, bleeding, and even ulcers. You can curtail these reactions by taking aspirin with milk or with a meal, taking antacids an hour after you take the aspirin, or using buffered or coated aspirin.

Aspirin can also cause dehydration. As you exercise, your temperature rises. Aspirin works to lower your temperature by increasing perspiration. This increased loss of fluid may cause you to become dehydrated and tire more easily. When you take aspirin, drink plenty of fluids to prevent dehydration. Don't wait until you feel thirsty. By that time, you may already be dehydrated.

I do not recommend that you take aspirin on a regular basis. However, if you are in a period where your muscles are constantly sore when you exercise, you may safely take two aspirin before or immediately after you exercise for a few days.

COCAINE

I once polled more than 100 top runners, asking them, "If I could give you a special pill to make you an Olympic champion—but that could also kill you in a year—would you take it?" More than half said yes. This desire for a quick and easy way to improve athletic performance is all too common. Many sports enthusiasts turn to cocaine for its supposed athletics-enhancing properties, although such properties are an illusion.

Q *Can cocaine improve athletic performance?*

A Cocaine is a potent stimulant that can raise your aggressions and cause you to feel less pain. That description may make cocaine sound as if it would be helpful to an athlete. It's not. Cocaine may prevent you from making intelligent decisions about when to stop hard physical activity. It charges you up so you may have no fear. At the same time, it does not make you stronger, or faster, or improve endurance. So while you may think you're doing wonderfully, you may really be doing poorly and running the risk of serious injury as well.

Dr. William Pollin, former director of the National Institute on Drug Abuse, says cocaine "may be the most seductive, intense, and threatening drug we know." This seductiveness is experienced by some athletes who are so stimulated by the drug that they need to take a sleeping pill to fall asleep. In the morning, they wake up depressed from effects of the sleeping pill and find it difficult to get out of bed without taking more cocaine.

Besides the well-reported physical damage that cocaine can inflict on the blood vessels of the nose, the drug also is a serious risk to anyone with heart or blood-pressure problems because it makes the heart pump faster and raises blood pressure. During exercise the risk greatly increases.

Exercise and cocaine don't mix—one is good for you, the other isn't.

CORTISONE

Q *I have severe asthma and must take cortisone every day to help me breathe. Since starting on cortisone, though, I have gained a lot of weight. Is there anything I can do to keep me from adding unwanted pounds?*

A Fight extra weight the only effective way: eat less and exercise more.

Cortisone affects some people's weight because it directly affects the brain's appetite control center and makes you feel hungry. Most people respond to this stimulus and eat more often. Exercise can help you to eat less. Knowing this, you should now take extra care to restrict your food intake and exercise more.

DIURETICS

Q *Is it possible to exercise safely while taking diuretics?*

A *Diuretics* are drugs that act on the kidneys to speed the expulsion of salt and water from the body. People who take these drugs must take special precautions if they also follow a regular exercise program. These precautions include drinking plenty of water during exercise and eating and drinking potassium-rich foods such as fresh fruits and their juices after exercise to replace fluids and potassium lost while working out.

These people, whose reason for taking diuretics is usually high blood pressure or fluid retention, should also be careful not to become overly tired during workouts. If exhaustion or weakness begin to overwhelm them, they should stop exercising immediately.

A study at Ball State University performed on a group of marathon runners showed the serious effects diuretics can have on exercisers. After taking diuretics, the runners vigorously worked out on a treadmill. Within 50 minutes, every athlete had passed out from lack of water.

During exercise, body fluids are continually lost through perspiration, which prevents the body from overheating. Taking a diuretic may cause you to lose too much body fluid. If this happens, your temperature may rise suddenly and cause you to pass out from the heat.

Because the body is unable to retain its usual amount of fluids when diuretics are taken, the amount of blood circulating in the body can also decrease. This, in itself, can cause weakness and elevated body temperature.

In addition, when most diuretics act on the kidneys, they block the reabsorption of potassium in the body, depleting the body's supply of that mineral. A low blood potassium level can make you weak and tired and can even cause an irregular heartbeat. You can prevent potassium deficiency by eating fresh fruits or drinking their juices.

INDERAL

Q *I've read that some divers, ski jumpers, and pistol shooters take a drug called Inderal before competition. Does it help them and if it does, how does it work?*

A *Inderal* is a drug that can calm you down, slow your heart rate, steady your hand, and prevent precompetition jitters.

When you wait for an athletic event to start, your heart often races and you feel shaky. That's because precompetition anxiety causes your body to produce increased amounts of a stimulant called *adrenalin*. It makes your heart beat faster, widens certain blood vessels so that more blood is pumped to your muscles and brain, widens the tubes leading to your lungs, and can stimulate you to the point of shakiness.

Inderal and other drugs in the same group can blunt some of these responses. By slowing down the heart, it can help people with certain types of heart disease. By helping them to stop shaking, it can benefit people with certain types of nerve disorders.

Inderal does not interfere with your strength, speed, or ability to jump. But, it can tire you more quickly than you would without the drug, so it should not be used for sporting events that require endurance.

Because it helps calm you down, it is mostly used for athletes performing tasks that require extreme concentration such as archery or diving.

Whatever competitive athletic exercise you do, you should check with your physician before you consider using Inderal.

MARIJUANA

Q *Can smoking marijuana help my training?*

A You can do lots of things to improve athletic performance, but training on grass is not one of them.

Smoking marijuana will not make you a better athlete. It can tire you more quickly while you exercise and will increase the time it takes you to recover afterward.

Marijuana can damage your lungs and make them less efficient when they take in oxygen to be carried throughout your body. THC, the active ingredient in marijuana, attaches itself to the carbon particles in the inhaled marijuana smoke more tightly than nicotine attaches to the carbon in tobacco smoke. To pry THC from the carbon particles, part of the process that gets a smoker "high," you must suck harder, inhale deeper, and hold the smoke in the lungs longer. This extra work is tiring.

Since marijuana smoke is held in the lungs longer, it is 16 times more damaging to the lungs than tobacco. At the University of California at Los Angeles, Dr. Donald Tashkin found that people who smoke five marijuana cigarettes a day for 45 days suffer a significant reduction in lung function. Studies at the E.G.&G. Mason Research Institute of Worcester, Massachusetts, show that laboratory rats suffered severe lung damage after just 87 days of daily marijuana smoking.

THC has been shown to damage cell membranes and delay tissue healing. Since your muscles are injured slightly every time you exercise, the THC in marijuana could delay muscle healing after you exercise.

Studies conducted at the University of California at Santa Barbara show that smoking marijuana also makes your heart work harder. Your heart beats 20 percent faster after you smoke just one joint. So, if you combine marijuana and exercise, your heart may need more time to return to its resting rate.

TOBACCO

Chewing Tobacco

Q *My 12-year-old son is crazy about baseball and plays it all the time. He watches baseball games on television and notices that most of the players chew tobacco. Now he's chewing tobacco because he thinks it will make him a better player. Why do they use it?*

A Baseball players probably chew tobacco because of the

nicotine in it. Nicotine, a stimulant, makes your heart beat faster and it makes you more alert when you feel tired.

There is no evidence that chewing tobacco will make you stronger, faster, better coordinated, or have greater endurance. Chewing tobacco is a dirty, unhealthy habit that increases your chances of developing mouth cancer, causes bad breath, discolors your teeth, impairs your ability to taste and smell, and can damage your gums. It's also just as addictive as smoking.

And, while baseball players can spit on the ground, your son will find he'll be a social outcast if he goes around spitting tobacco juice in public.

Smoking Tobacco

Q *If I start exercising will I be able to stop smoking?*

A An exercise regimen can help you stop cigarette smoking. Although exercise itself will not actually break the habit, it will keep the jittery smoker busy and away from cigarettes and it can help raise his or her mood. This is important for smokers, who frequently suffer depression while trying to kick their addiction to tobacco and its poisonous ingredient, nicotine.

No one really understands how exercise improves a person's mood, but most physicians believe it is due to the hormone norepinephrine, which is known to make people feel good. During exercise, your body releases increased amounts of this hormone.

Cigarette smoke contains large amounts of nicotine. Within eight seconds after inhaling cigarette smoke, a large concentration of the nicotine in that puff reaches your brain. The nicotine, which enters the brain directly from the bloodstream, triggers the release of hormones that cause your heart to beat faster than normal and your blood pressure to rise. This, unlikely as it may sound, calms you down and increases your ability to concentrate.

Shortly afterward, though, the nicotine level in your blood begins to drop and withdrawal symptoms develop. You may feel jittery and nervous and crave another cigarette. You may also get depressed.

Thus, a vicious cycle is under way. Each puff of a cigarette makes you feel relaxed, but you eventually grow jittery as the level of nicotine in your blood drops. You then smoke another cigarette to pick you up and you're on your way to a bad habit.

Once you've decided to quit, though, regular exercise can aid your success.

Marathons and Smoking

Q *I run marathons and smoke a pack of cigarettes a day. My best marathon time is 2 hours 40 minutes. How much faster would I run if I didn't smoke?*

A There is no exact answer to your question, but I can give you an approximate one.

How fast marathon runners are able to run depends on how quickly their muscles can withdraw oxygen from the bloodstream. The more oxygen they use, the faster they can run.

Oxygen is carried by red blood cells. The amount of oxygen your blood can carry is determined by the ability of your red blood cells to pick up and carry oxygen through your bloodstream. Smoking increases the amount of carbon monoxide in your body. In nonsmokers, about 1 to 2 percent of their red blood cells are bound by carbon monoxide. A recent study has demonstrated that in a pack-a-day smoker, 7 percent of his or her red blood cells are bound by carbon monoxide. That means that although the oxygen is in your bloodstream, 7 percent of your red blood cells cannot bind oxygen because they're already bound by carbon monoxide.

Therefore, you can expect a 7 percent reduction in your racing time. Seven percent of 160 minutes, your current racing time, equals a loss of 10 minutes.

Breathing Someone Else's Smoke

Q *I run 30 to 40 miles a week and at work I sit next to a four-pack-a-day smoker. Can this be harmful to me?*

A Yes, breathing someone else's smoke can be harmful to you. At least two recent studies show that over a period of years, breathing other people's smoke may cause damage to the small air tubes that lead to the air sacs in your lungs.

Smoke causes damage to the *cilia*, hairlike organisms that sweep mucus out of your lungs. The more cilia that are damaged, the more difficult it is to expel mucus out of your lungs, which is why people with emphysema cough so much.

You have legal recourse against smokers at work. Several successful lawsuits have forced owners to protect workers from factors that will harm their health at work.

If you would like instructions on what you can do if you are forced to breathe other people's smoke, send a contribution and a request to:

> Action On Smoking And Health
> 2000 H Street, N.W.
> Washington, D.C. 20006

TRANQUILIZERS

Q *My doctor has suggested that he could prescribe tranquilizers to help me cope with nervousness and anxiety. How will these drugs affect me when I exercise?*

AAs tranquilizers calm you down, they generally slow you down as well. To do that, they decrease the electrical activity in your brain, which causes you to tire more easily. In general, they can diminish your endurance and interfere with your coordination while exercising.

There are four major types of tranquilizers, each with its own side effects. One group treats thought disorders such as schizophrenia, another treats depression, a third treats the mania that is characterized by an unrealistically high emotional state, and a fourth group is used to treat anxiety.

Haldol, Thorazine, and Compazine are common drugs for treating thought disorders. These drugs can interfere with your coordination and make you very tired.

Common antidepressants include Elavil and Sinequan, which can cause irregular heartbeats during exercise. They can also make you dizzy. For people with heart disease, this can be dangerous. For others it will probably be mildly bothersome.

Lithium is the best and most frequently used drug to treat people who are manic. It can interfere with coordination and drain fluid from your body so that you are more likely to become dehydrated when you exercise while using Lithium.

The most frequently used prescription drug in the United States today is Valium, which, along with Librium, is used to treat anxiety. Both of these tranquilizers can cause tiredness and weakness.

All of these tranquilizers can affect your athletic performance, making it difficult for you to pitch a well-placed baseball, get the basketball in the basket or play a strong game of tennis.

If you notice any of the side effects mentioned, check with your physician to see whether your dose should be changed or you should switch to another medication. Usually, a physician will recommend lowering the dosage.

10
ISSUES RELATED TO EXERCISING IN HOT AND COLD WEATHER

DRESSING FOR THE COLD

Several years ago a young couple wearing blue jeans and denim jackets were caught in a rainstorm while jogging along the Appalachian Trail. They both died of low body temperature, or *hypothermia*, even though the outside temperature never went below 38°F.

The blue jeans and denim jackets, which were both made of cotton, lost more than 95 percent of their insulating properties when wet. Wearing wet cotton clothes, the joggers had little more protection than they would have had they went naked.

You need to be well-prepared when you exercise in cold weather, and *layering*, wearing several layers of clothing to remove or put on according to changes in the weather and your level of activity, is the best way to do that.

A heavy outer garment is unnecessary because insulation is determined by the thickness of the garment, not by its weight. The more layers you put on, the more air is trapped. And, air is an excellent insulator; it allows you to retain your body heat.

Q *What is the best outerwear to use when exercising in cold weather?*

A The best outer layers are those made of tightly woven fibers such as wool or nylon, which block wind and rain. The worst fiber for outer garments when you exercise in cold weather is cotton.

For the middle and inner layers, use materials that insulate well and carry perspiration rapidly away from your body so it doesn't cool you. Loosely woven fibers made of nylon and polyester are ideal.

Contrary to what you may have heard, cotton is a very poor material to wear next to your skin in winter because it absorbs perspiration and holds it against your skin, which may cool your body to dangerously low levels.

KEEPING WARM

Q *Why. do hats, socks, and gloves protect you better against cold than any other garments?*

A Remember when you were a child and your mother told you never to go out in cold weather without your mittens, hat, and warm socks? Well, mother was right. To protect yourself when you exercise in cold weather, you should keep your fingers, head, and toes warm.

You feel the cold through nerve receptors in your skin, not from your lowered body temperature. The most sensitive receptors for cold are in your fingers, ears, head, and toes. As long as they are warm, you'll feel warm.

To protect your hands, wear mittens, not gloves, which allow the individual fingers to warm each other. The best mittens have an inner material to draw the perspiration away from your skin, and an outer material that will not lose its insulating properties when wet. Silk is an ideal inner material, because it rapidly wicks perspiration away from your skin. Wool is an excellent outer material because it dries from the inside out, retaining its insulating ability even when wet.

You lose heat more quickly from your head than from any other part of your body. When you feel cold, your body responds by closing its blood vessels. But, because there are numerous blood vessels on your scalp, they don't constrict as well as those in other parts of your body. The colder it gets outside, the more heat you lose through your head, because the blood vessels in the rest of your body will have already constricted. For example, at 20°F, more than 40 percent of your heat loss is through your head; at 5°F, that figure increases to 70 percent.

On moderately cold days, it's enough to wear a woolen ski hat that pulls down over your ears. On very cold days—below 32°F—you should also wear a hood to cover your neck.

As for your feet, wear thick woolen socks and warm, padded, well-fitting boots when you're doing any outdoor exercise other than running. When you run, you generate enough heat naturally so you'll be warm enough wearing your regular running shoes.

ACCLIMATIZATION TO COLD

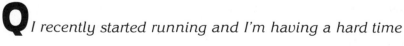 **Q** *I recently started running and I'm having a hard time*

adjusting to the cold weather. Will I ever adapt?

A Many runners dread the onset of winter. But, as they are repeatedly exposed to colder temperatures during their regular runs, they find they don't mind it as much.

The most likely explanation for this gradual adaptation to the cold is the fact that exposure to low temperatures causes your body to make more brown fat cells that are sensitive to norepinephrine, a hormone that induces fat to produce more heat.

There are two types of fat in your body—yellow and brown. More than 99 percent is yellow fat, located under your skin and around your major organs. A smaller amount is brown fat, located between your shoulder blades, in your armpits, and around the blood vessels leading to your heart and kidneys.

The heat-producing brown fat around the vessels leading to your heart is very important in protecting you from the winter weather. When you exercise in the cold, the blood in your arms, legs, and head cools. Brown fat in your chest warms that blood as it returns to your heart. If cold blood ever reaches that organ, it can cause irregular heartbeats and even death.

Keep up your cold weather exercise. You eventually will adapt and you'll look forward to your brisk winter runs.

SHOVELING SNOW

Q *Is it true that shoveling snow can be fatal?*

A A 63-year-old man in Minnesota recently suffered a fatal heart attack while shoveling snow from his driveway. Incidents like this occur every winter because shoveling snow is a strain on the heart.

Researchers in Toronto report that the exertion of shoveling snow, not the low temperature, is the culprit in winter-related heart attack victims and discovered that most attacks occur on the day after a snowfall, not necessarily on the coldest days.

Wet snow is very heavy. When you shovel it, your heart has to work 2½ times as hard to pump blood through your arms as it does to pump the same amount through your legs. Muscles and blood vessels in your arms are smaller than those in your legs, creating greater resistance against blood flow.

Q *How can I shovel snow safely even though I'm not in the best of shape?*

A If you are out-of-shape and become short of breath when you walk briskly, your heart may be too weak for you to lift a snow-filled shovel safely. Your heart will struggle to supply blood to your arms and you may develop an irregular heartbeat. You could even suffer a heart attack.

When shoveling snow this winter, remember to:

- fill the shovel only halfway.
- hold the shovel close to your body to make it easier to lift.
- bend your knees when you reach down for the snow and rise by straightening your knees to put less strain on your arms and protect your heart.

If you have not been exercising much, you can do simple exercises to strengthen your heart and arms. Especially good for your heart are riding a stationary bicycle, jogging in place, walking rapidly, and pulling on a rowing machine.

To strengthen your arms, lifting barbells can be specifically tailored for shoveling snow. Hold a lightweight barbell (25 pounds) at thigh height, with palms forward and elbows straight. Imitate the shoveling motion by bending your knees. Then, while straightening them, slowly raise the barbell to your shoulder. Do three sets (10 times each) of this exercise daily, resting a minute between each set. Increase the weight of the barbell as your arms become stronger.

BREATHING THROUGH YOUR NOSE

Q *Is it advisable to breathe only through my nose during cold weather to avoid unpleasant effects of cold air on the mouth?*

A Don't try to breathe only through your nose when exercising in cold weather.

Your nose does help warm the air you breathe, but its openings are so small that when you pick up the pace you won't get enough oxygen and may turn blue.

During exercise you need plenty of oxygen. The amount of air you inhale depends on the size of the passageways leading to the lungs. The cross-sectional area of your nasal openings is less than one-tenth that of your throat. You won't be able to take in enough oxygen through your nose alone to supply your body during hard exercise. You're better off breathing through your mouth.

Some people are concerned about breathing very cold air through their mouths. They fear a mythical condition known as *frozen lungs*. It is almost impossible to damage your lungs by inhaling cold air. During exercise your body markedly increases its heat production. The extra heat warms the air that you breathe in. For example, air taken in at minus 40°F will be warmed to almost 100°F before it reaches your lungs. Besides, you probably will never face that situation because inhaling air that cold would be so painful to your nose and throat that you would quickly lose interest in outdoor exercise and seek shelter.

If breathing in frigid air while you exercise makes you uncomfortable, try wearing a face mask that covers both your mouth and nose. It looks very much like the protective masks industrial painters use when spraying heavy machinery. The mask is porous enough to let the air in and out, yet solid enough to help you retain heat and moisture. Such masks usually can be purchased at sporting-goods stores, especially ski shops and other outlets devoted to winter activities.

ACCLIMATIZATION TO HEAT

Q *Are there any special methods of preparing for exercise in a hot climate?*

A It is very important to prepare yourself for exercising in hot weather. You can still do as much as you usually do. Nevertheless, you need to pay attention to what your body may be telling you about overheating. If you ignore certain distress signals, your body temperature may rise too high, which can heat your brain cells enough for you to pass out and perhaps even die.

The process of preparing your body to withstand the heat so that your body temperature won't rise uncontrollably is called *acclimatization*. This process involves training your heart to become more effective at pumping blood through your body. When you exercise in the heat, your heart must pump a markedly increased amount of blood from your heated muscles to the skin, where the heat is dissipated. Muscle temperatures of up to 107°F are not unusual during exercise in hot weather.

How do you acclimatize? By exercising with caution, paying attention to such body signals as unusual pounding of your heart, unexplained shortness of breath, headache, dizziness, or extreme fatigue. If you notice any of these symptoms, stop exercising and rest until the following day.

Q *How long will it take for my body to adjust to exercising in the heat this summer?*

A It takes 4 to 14 days for your body to adjust to the heat; the sweat glands in your skin must become enlarged so you can sweat more and your blood vessels must widen so that your body will be able to send large amounts of blood to your skin. This is necessary because when you exercise, your body produces tremendous amounts of heat. If your body cannot get rid of that extra heat, your temperature can rise high enough to cause you to faint.

Your body acclimates to the heat only if you exercise in the heat. Lying on the beach will not prepare you for exercising in the heat. Neither will living in a hot climate unless you also exercise outdoors. In fact, you can acclimatize to the heat even in a cold climate. All you must do is exercise wearing enough clothing to make you perspire heavily. For example, the 1964 U.S. Olympic Marathon trials were run at noon in New York in 100°F heat. Buddy Edelin, who lives in chilly England, won the race by more than 20 minutes. Edelin had acclimatized his body to the heat by training while wearing five sweat suits!

The best advice is to take it easy the first few days you

exercise in hot weather and allow your body to adapt at its own rate.

SLOWER IN THE HEAT

Q *Why are the winning times in roadrunning races slower in the summer?*

A In hot weather the heart has to work much harder to cool the body. Only 30 percent of the energy produced by the body is used to power your muscles; the other 70 percent is used to produce heat. This heat, which increases during exercise, must be dissipated to the skin. The heart does this by pumping large amounts of blood from the hot muscles to the skin, where the heat is released. People who run in road races during hot weather are putting more of a strain on their hearts just to maintain normal body temperature, which slows down the efficiency of their muscles and their running speed. Hot weather can be dangerous for healthy road runners, but for people with weak hearts, running in hot weather can be fatal.

SALT TABLETS

Q *I run every day even when the weather is very hot. I know that I lose a lot of salt in my sweat. Should I take salt tablets?*

A There are two reasons why you shouldn't take salt tablets.

First, the American diet is loaded with so much salt that most of us get far more than we need. The average American takes in between 6,000 and 18,000 milligrams of salt per day. When you exercise in hot weather, you need only around 3,000.

And second, if you take salt tablets when you don't need them, you can develop a high blood concentration of salt, which is more harmful than having too little. High blood levels of salt increase the chance of clots forming in your blood vessels. Salt can also act on your kidneys to prevent your kidney tubules from reabsorbing water; you lose more water and can become dehydrated. This will make you weak and tired and can increase your chances of passing out when you exercise.

If you exercise in the heat and feel weak and tired or develop muscle cramps, check with your doctor. A simple blood test will determine if you lack salt. If the blood test is normal, you need to find another explanation for your tiredness or cramps. If your blood salt level is low, you may need to add more salt to your food.

DRINKING DURING HOT WEATHER

Q *When and how much should I drink if I exercise in hot weather? Won't I get cramps if I drink too much?*

A A few years ago, a coach in the National Football League wouldn't let his players drink during hot weather practice. Five of his players, including his starting quarterback, ended up in the hospital because of *heat stroke*, a sudden rise in body temperature that can cause you to pass out. Nowadays, we recommend that all people drink fluid when they exercise in hot weather.

When you exercise, your temperature will start to rise. Your body responds by producing sweat, which evaporates from your skin and cools your body. During vigorous exercise, you can lose 5 pints or 5 pounds of sweat per hour. When you lose 3 percent of your body weight through sweat, your body temperature will start to rise and you will become weaker, slower, and feel tired. A 150-pound man who exercises vigorously in hot weather can lose 3 percent of his weight or 4½ pounds in an hour. Once you have lost that much fluid, no matter how much you drink, you will not be able to catch up on your fluid loss during exercise.

So, on hot days, drink a cup of cold water just before you start to exercise. Cold water is absorbed more rapidly than warm water and is less likely to cause stomach cramps. It causes your stomach to contract and push the water into your intestines where the water is absorbed immediately. You should also try to drink water at least every 15 minutes while you exercise.

When you exercise continuously for less than 2½ hours, you usually won't need to take in any minerals and you won't need to take in any extra calories.

INDEX